P9-EMK-860

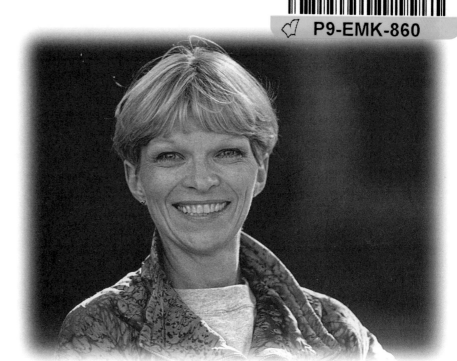

*H*ello—

I'm Terrie Rizzo.
I work at the
Stanford Center
for Research in Disease Prevention with
some of the world's leading experts in exercise
and health promotion. We've developed
Fresh Start to help people like you, who want to
become fitter, trimmer, and healthier—for life.

You can begin today to make a fresh start. It
doesn't matter if you've never exercised before,
or you haven't exercised in a long time: You can
start today and see your health and vitality
improve surprisingly quickly.

In our programs we've seen thousands of people of all sizes and ages who never dreamed they could become fit achieve their goals.

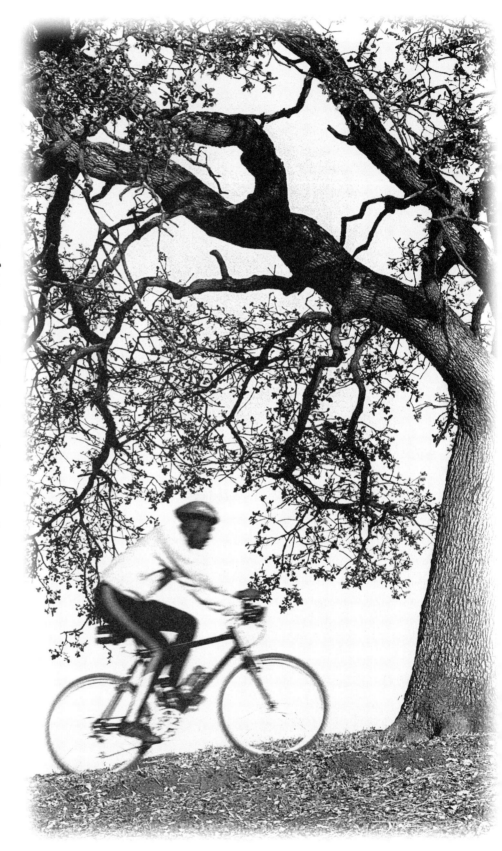

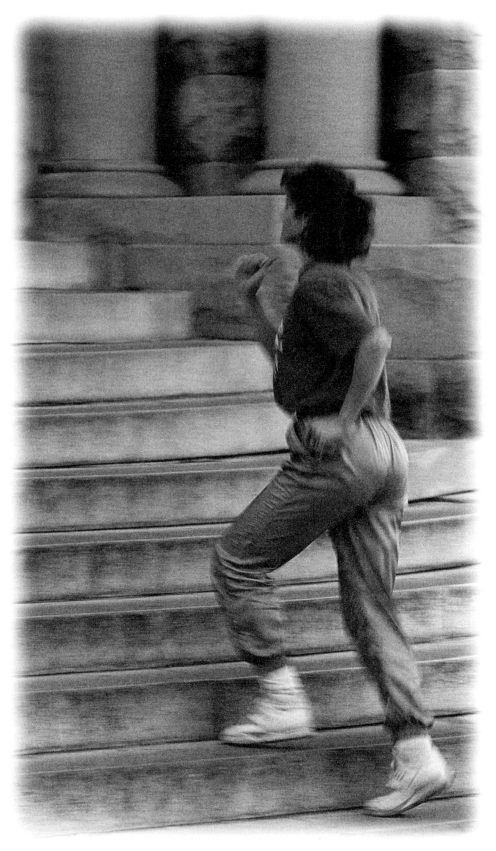

With regular, moderate-intensity exercise, doing activities that you enjoy and look forward to, you can add years to your life and life to your years.

*B*egin today to enjoy a...

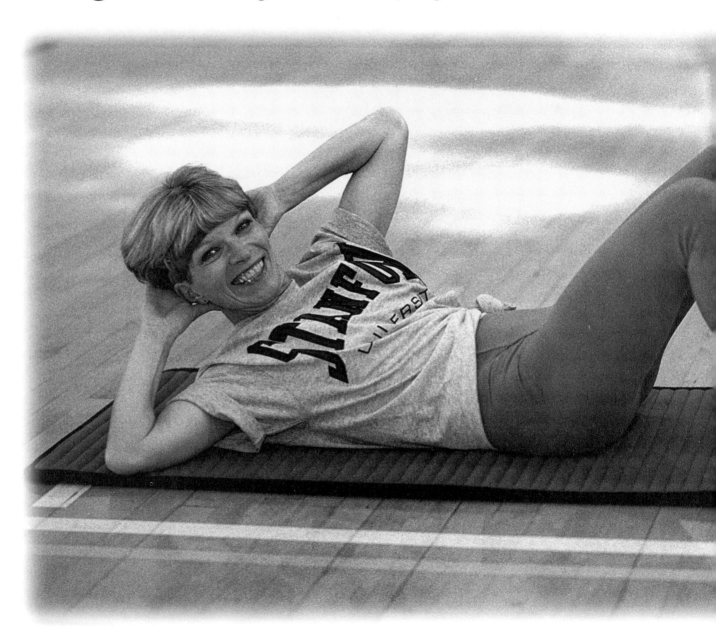

Fresh Start

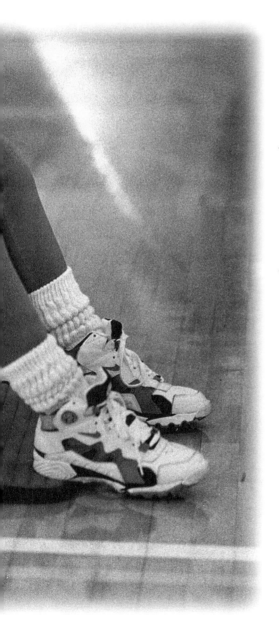

The Stanford Medical School
Health and Fitness Program

*Developed by the Stanford Center
for Research in Disease Prevention
in partnership with the
Stanford Alumni Association*

Foreword by Wesley F. Alles, PH.D.
Introduction by John W. Farquhar, M.D.

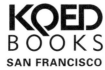

KQED
BOOKS
SAN FRANCISCO

© 1996 by Stanford Alumni Association and the Board of Trustees of the
Leland Stanford Jr. University.

All rights reserved.

No part of this book may be used or reproduced in any manner whatsoever
without the written permission of the Publisher, except in the case of brief
quotations in critical articles and reviews. For information, address:
KQED Books & Video, 2601 Mariposa St., San Francisco, CA 94110.

Vice President for Publishing & New Ventures: Mark K. Powelson

PUBLISHER: Pamela Byers
MANAGING EDITOR: Sheryl Fullerton
CONSULTING EDITOR: Michael Castleman
EDITOR: Naomi Lucks
BOOK DESIGN AND ART DIRECTION: Paula Schlosser
PHOTOGRAPHER: Nita Winter
PRODUCTION DIRECTOR: Brad Stauffer
PRINT PRODUCTION COORDINATOR: Ellen Reese
FOR STANFORD ALUMNI ASSOCIATION: Catherine O'Brien

KQED President & CEO: Mary G. F. Bitterman

Educational and non-profit groups wishing to order this book at attractive
quantity discounts may contact KQED Books & Video, 2601 Mariposa St.,
San Francisco, CA 94110.

Earlier versions of Chapters 1, 2, 3, 5, 6, 7, 9, 13, 14, and 17 appeared in
The Stanford Health & Exercise Handbook by the Stanford Alumni Association
with the Stanford Center for Research in Disease Prevention, © 1987.

LIBRARY OF CONGRESS CATALOGUING-IN-PUBLICATION DATA
Fresh Start: the Stanford Medical School health and fitness program/developed by the Stanford Center for Research in Disease Prevention in partnership with the Stanford Alumni Association: foreword by Jack Farquhar: preface by Terrie Heinrich Rizzo.
  p. cm.
Portions previously published as: The Stanford Health & Exercise Handbook. Stanford, CA, 1987.
Includes bibliographical references and index.
    ISBN 0-912333-33-2 (pbk.)
    1. Exercise. 2. Health.
    I. Stanford Center for Research in Disease Prevention.
    II. Stanford Alumni Association.
RA781.F685 1996
613.7—dc20   95-26735   CIP

ISBN 0-912333-33-2

Manufactured in the United States of America

10 9 8 7 6 5 4 3 2 1

Distributed to the trade by Publishers Group West

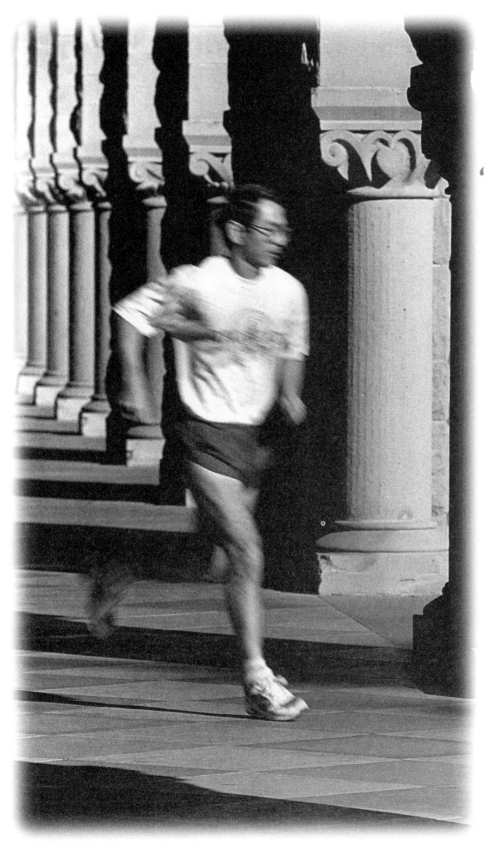

"This book is for real people, with real bodies, who want to look and feel better. Exercise absolutely is the key." —Terrie Rizzo

Contents

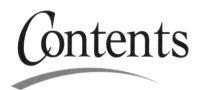

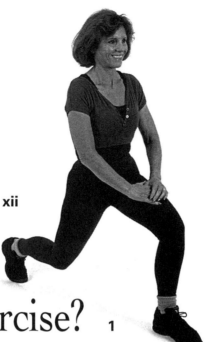

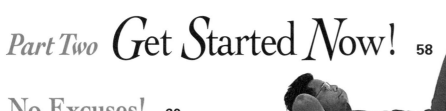

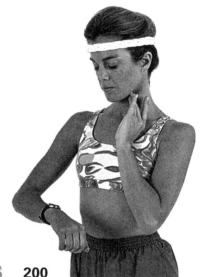

Foreword

Wesley F. Alles, PH.D.

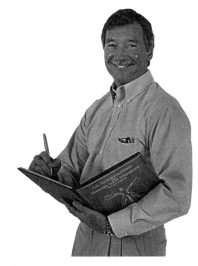

WHERE OUR HEALTH IS CONCERNED, the phrase "An ounce of prevention is worth a pound of cure" has never been more true. The decisions that we make every day about exercise, nutrition, weight management, smoking, and stress have a direct influence on our susceptibility to heart disease and stroke, many types of cancer, diabetes, and other chronic conditions. For most of us, making just a few important changes in our lives will dramatically alter our risk of illness and improve our quality of life. And that is what this book is all about.

The Stanford Center for Research in Disease Prevention (originally called the Stanford Heart Disease Prevention Program) was begun in 1971 under the direction of John W. Farquhar, M.D. Here professionals from such diverse fields as medicine, public health, the behavioral sciences, health communication, lipidology (the study of fats), nutrition, exercise physiology, and health education conduct extensive research efforts, test the effectiveness of various prevention and education strategies, and develop materials that enable other professionals and the public to benefit from the research.

The information in this book represents the very latest research into health promotion and disease prevention. Each chapter was written by doctors and health professionals who are experts in their fields. But the information alone won't change your life: You will benefit only if you follow the recommended guidelines. If you need help, talk with your primary care physician or check with your health plan.

As far as your health goes, there's no time like the present to begin!

Wesley F. Alles, PH.D., is the Director of the Stanford Health Improvement Program and Senior Research Scientist at the SCRDP. He exercises five times a week—four days jogging and one day weight-lifting.

As far as your health goes, there's no time like the present to begin!

*I*ntroduction

John W. Farquhar, M.D.

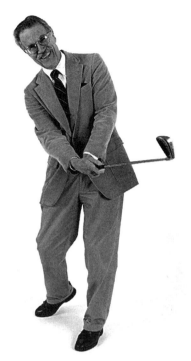

John W. Farquhar, M.D., is the Director of the Stanford Center for Research in Disease Prevention. He is Professor of Medicine, Professor of Health Research and Policy, and the C. F. Rehnborg Professor of Disease Prevention. His program of exercise includes regular circuit weight training and stationary cycling, and he also enjoys hiking, kayaking, and canoeing whenever possible.

WE SHOULD ALL HOPE FOR one blessing: to live out our allotted life span in peace, freedom, dignity, and health. When we become ill, our quality of life is reduced and our productivity is limited. Anyone whose hair is turning gray knows that health, as a personal commodity, grows in value with age.

Nonetheless, in my thirty years as a physician, I have never ceased to be amazed at the abuse inflicted indifferently or deliberately on the human body. We tend to ignore our responsibility for its maintenance and the consequences of our actions. We assume—perhaps arrogantly, perhaps hopefully—that illness will happen to someone else, while never to ourselves.

Today we know that habits and lifestyle influence our health, that what we are born with is not what we will die with. Along the way from birth to death, our arteries get clogged, our lungs polluted, our organs diseased, our muscles atrophied. Yet we can prevent many of these things from happening with just a modicum of effort.

Health is a natural resource, and we should make every effort to preserve it. Most of us are born into this world as perfect human specimens; but long before we leave this world, our packaging and performance change for the worse. We are beset with all the problems that flesh is heir to. Is this march toward illness and decrepitude inevitable, or can we do something to prevent our own obsolescence?

What threatens us today is different from the massive cripplers and killers in history—bubonic plague, cholera, or polio. Our number-one killer and our number-one health problem—the smallpox of this generation—is cardiovascular disease. It kills 700,000 people a year from heart attack and strokes, and seriously afflicts another 1 million people each year with pain and disability.

But unlike smallpox and similar dread diseases, cardiovascular disease, certain cancers, emphysema, and adult-onset diabetes are products of the risks incurred by living in the industrialized twentieth century. The inoculation we need for protection against these diseases is not the prick of a needle, but rather a change in our thinking.

What happens to our bodies as we move through life is the result of our habits, the bits and pieces of the way we live. We are what we do; we become what we have done.

Sigmund Freud said that the ultimate purpose of life was to love and to work. I would add that one also needs to be in good health. When you have love, work, and health, you have made a place for yourself in the world and you enhance the world.

Maintaining good health while pursuing love and work is the task of the wise man and woman. The goal is to be and remain optimally healthy for as long as possible, and to exit gracefully.

Good health is priceless—and, paradoxically, it is freely available to us if we live the right way. The child does not have to be taught to play, but the adult must learn how to exercise. Many of us on the road to adulthood lose that childhood instinct to run and jump, to skip with joy, to walk briskly through the crisp autumn leaves. But it is movement, in assorted styles and speeds, on a regular basis, that is critical to maintaining our astoundingly complicated and wonderful bodies.

In the recent past, most people got their exercise easily, through the tasks of daily living. Before automobiles and elevators took our feet from the ground, we walked more. Our grandparents chopped wood and pitched hay. Women kneaded dough for bread, leaned over their washboards and scrubbed clothes. All were exercising. Today we live in a world where exercise is something that we must superimpose onto ordinary living.

I can give you eight good reasons for making the effort. It takes a bit of time, but the benefits are worth it:

- Your cardiovascular health will improve.
- You will keep your weight under control.
- You will increase your muscle mass and strength.
- You will lower your blood sugar.
- You will lower your blood pressure.
- You will increase your bone density.
- You will feel psychologically healthier.
- You will slow down the aging process.

Of these eight, the last two are the most difficult to measure but hold the greatest emotional reward. With faithful exercise, your sense of well-being and confidence improves. The better your self-image, through weight loss and muscle toning, the better you feel about yourself. You have a sense of energy and resilience. With that comes the feeling that you're holding back time. You are vigorous and energetic; you feel that you are living more each day; and your physician tells you that the pounds are indeed melting away, the cholesterol and blood pressure are dropping, and your heart functions today as it did fifteen years ago.

The best news is that it is never too late to start exercising. Regardless of your age or physical condition, you still have time to begin. In my own experience with patients, I have observed that it's never too late and it's never too early. This book can help you begin to make those changes that will sustain your health for life.

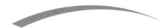

Good scholarship happens only with the excellent participation of all involved. For their generous time, effort, and enthusiasm, I wish to thank the staff and associates of the Stanford Center for Research in Disease Prevention, the Stanford Sports Medicine Department, and the Stanford Alumni Association. Additionally, I offer my thanks to James Fries, M.D., Professor of Medicine at the Stanford School of Medicine, for his very effective expression, "compressed morbidity"—a longer span of good health followed by a brief period of illness at the end of a full life.

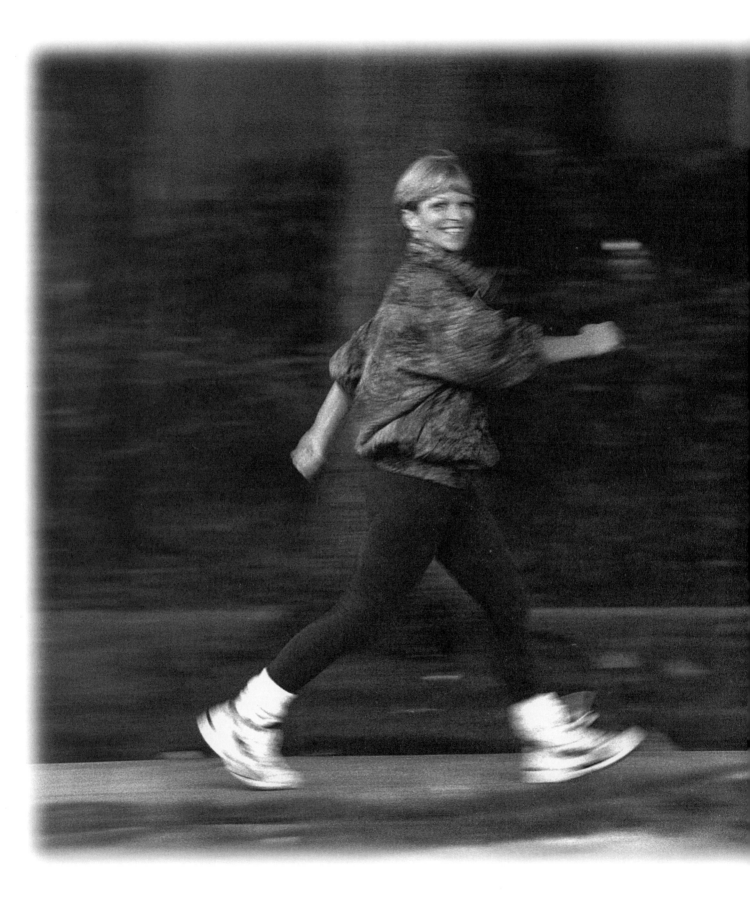

Part One

Why Exercise?

"Why exercise? The real question is, Why not exercise? Regular, moderate-intensity exercise can improve your health, your fitness, and your outlook on life. And everyone—regardless of sex, age, or athletic ability—can reap the benefits."

—Terrie Rizzo

Change
Your Life
with
Exercise

William L. Haskell, PH.D.

You have nothing to lose, and everything to gain, from adding exercise to your life. And it's never too soon—or too late— to start.

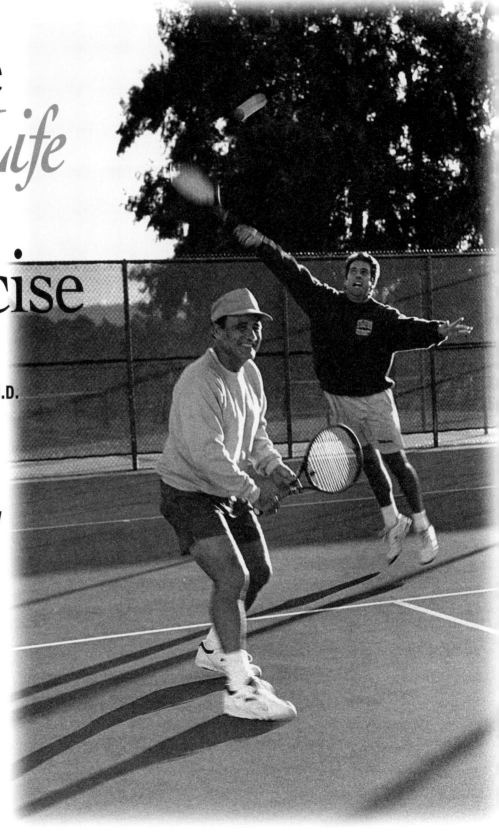

*S*O MANY EXTRAVAGANT CLAIMS have been made for exercise in recent years that many people have taken it up with misplaced expectations. Finding that exercise did not (as they had hoped) change their personality, improve their thinking processes, make them quit smoking, revolutionize their sex lives, fix their constipation, eliminate their wrinkles, and bring them an indefinable "high," they gave up—and thus deprived themselves of the very real and important benefits that exercise can indeed bring.

You don't need to run marathons or even ten-kilometer races to achieve the many health and performance benefits of exercise. We now have ample evidence that they can be attained at levels of exercise that are well within the capacity of most people. For example, studies have shown that people who are more active have a lower risk of heart attacks or adult-onset diabetes—even when their exercise consisted mostly of gardening, stair climbing, vigorous walking, or active sports.

How does exercise reduce this risk? When metabolism shifts to a higher gear to supply the increase in energy needed during exercise, the body undergoes a number of changes designed to help the muscles work more efficiently, increase their capacity, and reduce fatigue. The various systems in the body that support and supply the muscles respond to the need for extra work by increasing their capacity and becoming more efficient. Thus exercise has a beneficial effect on your muscles, nervous system, cardiovascular system, respiratory system, and bones, and makes the way you burn fats and carbohydrates more efficient.

When you combine a good exercise program with other good health habits—like eating a low-fat, high-complex carbo-

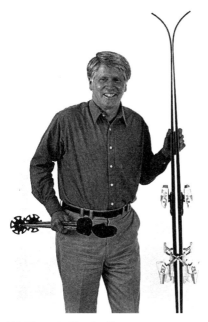

William L. Haskell, PH.D., is Professor of Medicine at Stanford University School of Medicine, Deputy Director of SCRDP, consultant to the President's Council on Physical Fitness and Sports, and past President of the American College of Sports Medicine. He participates in a variety of activities, including jogging, hiking, and skiing.

Nine Benefits of Exercise

1. It improves the health of your cardiovascular system.

2. It helps you control your weight.

3. It builds lean muscles.

4. It improves blood fat and cholesterol profiles.

5. It improves glucose (sugar) metabolism.

6. It helps lower blood pressure.

7. It maintains and even increases bone density.

8. It improves psychological health.

9. It slows the aging process.

hydrate diet and not smoking—it can provide highly significant health benefits that affect both body and mind.

Exercise Improves Cardiovascular Health

Exercise has a striking affect on coronary heart disease. Studies over the past decade show that men and women who are routinely physically active are far less likely to die of coronary artery disease—the cause of most heart attacks—than people who are sedentary. This benefit is independent of other heart disease risk factors, which means that being active provides protection beyond just being lean or having a normal cholesterol or blood pressure level.

Physical exercise helps control other risk factors, such as obesity, blood pressure, and cholesterol levels. What's more, regular exercise may have a direct effect on the coronary arteries that makes them healthier and better able to respond to the stresses of life. For more on this subject, read the chapter on Exercising After a Heart Attack.

A wide variety of activities seems to provide benefit, especially all forms of aerobic activity. The best program for cardiac health is a schedule of aerobic activities of moderate intensity that lasts thirty minutes or more, performed on most days. See Get Moving, Keep Moving—Aerobically for information.

Exercise Helps Keep Off Weight

Exercise has a wonderful ability to help control body weight. In fact, many people find it difficult to control their weight without exercise.

For example, a small-boned woman who is inactive can maintain her weight by eating no more than 1,200 calories a day. To lose weight by diet alone, she would have to eat far less, and would probably find it extremely difficult to maintain a sufficient intake of nutrients while eating so little food. Clearly, it makes sense for her to expend a few hundred additional calories in exercise so that she can eat more. An exercise program that uses up only an additional 200 to 300 calories a day would allow her to increase her calorie intake by 20 percent and still not gain weight. For more on diet and exercise, see the chapter Eat Well, Be Well.

Exercise Helps Build Good-Quality Muscles

When we talk about muscle mass, it really is a case of "Use it or lose it." If we use our muscles, they stay strong. If we don't, they grow weak—no matter how old we are, or what kind of shape we're in.

Without good-quality muscles, every physical action becomes more of an effort. We need good muscles to walk to the store, carry groceries, climb the stairs to the bedroom, balance on the stepladder to change a light bulb . . . the list is virtually endless. If you allow your muscles to deteriorate as you grow older, you will be less well equipped to care for yourself later in life. Since many Americans are now living well into their seventies and eighties, maintaining muscle strength by regular exercise has become essential for self-reliance and quality of life.

Muscle requires more calories for its normal maintenance than does fat tissue. This means that if you develop and main-

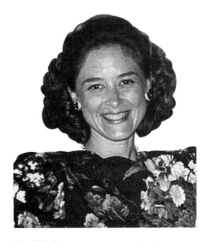

Tia Rich, M.A., M.S.W., is the former Assistant Director of the Stanford Health Improvement Program. A Ph.D. candidate at U.C. Berkeley, she conducts research and training programs on the prevention and management of stress, particularly occupational stress. She is the author of the "Myths and Facts" which appear throughout *Fresh Start*.

Myth: **Exercise increases your risk of pulling a muscle or hurting your knees or back.**

Fact: **The greatest risk of exercise is *not* doing it. When you follow recommended guidelines, exercise increases the body's overall functioning and actually helps to protect from illness and injury.**

tain a good proportion of muscle mass rather than fat, you will find it easier to control your weight. Simply put, at the same body weight, you can eat more without gaining weight if your weight is more muscle than fat. For more details, see the chapters Why Exercise Works and Using Your Muscles for Life.

Exercise Builds Bone and Retards Osteoporosis

Exercise can play an important role in helping to prevent bone fractures due to osteoporosis—loss of bone density—in post-menopausal women and older men. Any activity that applies force to bone will help build or maintain bone density.

Fortunately, you don't have to be an athlete to reap the benefits. All of the aerobic activities advocated throughout this book—such as running, walking, dancing, bicycling, or stair climbing, and resistance exercises like weight training, help build or maintain bone density, especially of the legs, hips, and back.

Ideally, your exercise habit should begin in childhood and adolescence, when increased stress on the developing bones will cause more calcium to be added to them, providing reserves that will be valuable later in life when mineral loss starts to occur. But it's virtually never too late to start.

Exercise has also been shown to slow the rate of bone mineral loss in postmenopausal women. A Wisconsin study compared two groups of older women. The first group exercised three times a week for thirty minutes each session, and the other group was sedentary. The results were striking: The

Myth: It doesn't matter what I do—middle-aged spread is inevitable.

Fact: Wrong! Regular exercise helps prevent "natural" age-related weight gain—millions of exercisers are successfully fighting the battle of the bulge.

women who exercised showed a net gain in bone density of 2.3 percent, while the non-exercisers showed an average bone mineral loss of 3.3 percent over the same period.

No one knows precisely how much exercise is needed to retain bone mineral content, but it is clear that the less active we are, the more calcium we lose. People who are confined to bed will lose calcium much more rapidly than those who do even a minimal amount of weight-bearing activity. In short, any exercise is better than no exercise, and systematic activity can plainly be of value.

Frequent exercise may also help prevent bone fractures by reducing the risk of injurious falls. New evidence demonstrates that exercise programs that build strength, endurance, and flexibility help prevent older people from falling. Also, stronger muscles may help protect bones during a fall.

Swimming Builds Bones, Too

Swimming may not seem like a weight-bearing exercise, but a study by Dr. Eric S. Orwoll, a Portland, Oregon, endocrinologist, suggests that swimming can also prevent calcium loss to the bones.

Dr. Orwoll studied fifty-eight men over forty who had been swimming for at least three hours a week for at least three years. All were nonsmokers who drank little alcohol, and swimming was their only sport. He found that the swimmers' bones had substantially more calcium than those of seventy-eight nonexercising men in the same age group who followed the same diet.

This could be good news for people concerned about osteoporosis—especially those who must avoid weight-bearing exercises, or who just like to swim.

Exercise Helps Process Carbohydrates and Insulin

Frequent exercise at moderate intensity may significantly contribute to a reduced risk of adult-onset diabetes—the type of diabetes that usually occurs after age thirty-five and is an increasingly common disorder in older men and women. In two large studies, fewer of those who exercised at least two or three times per week developed diabetes than people who were sedentary.

It now appears that frequent exercise, combined with leanness, significantly contribute to a reduced risk of diabetes later in life. Some people who already have diabetes can effectively manage their disease by exercising regularly and keeping their fat weight down.

Exercise can do this because it has a direct effect on carbohydrates and insulin. Regular exercise enhances the way the body processes carbohydrates. During large-muscle exercise of moderate intensity, the body uses glycogen stored in the muscles to produce energy. For several days after the stored glycogen is depleted, it is replaced by glucose in the blood.

Exercise also reduces the body's need for insulin by increasing its insulin sensitivity. One study compared the blood of exercisers and nonexercisers right after meals, when the circulating glucose is at its height and the body increases the output of insulin to deal with that glucose. Researchers found that the nonexercisers required twice as much insulin as the exercisers to remove glucose from their blood.

Myth: You need to do intense aerobic activity at least three times a week to get the benefits of exercise.

Fact: All physical activity is beneficial. It is as important for your health to regularly move through a full range of motion as it is to work up a heart-thumping, deep-breathing sweat!

Exercise Helps Balance Cholesterol Levels

Exercise directly affects the cholesterol balance of the blood by increasing levels of the beneficial type (high-density-lipoprotein cholesterol, or HDL). Many studies have shown that athletes such as marathon runners, cross-country runners, and dedicated tennis players have much higher levels of beneficial HDL cholesterol and lower triglycerides than nonexercisers.

> "Exercise makes you feel good in so many ways. At first you may find it difficult, but very soon you'll begin to feel the many benefits that come from physical activity."
>
> —Terrie Rizzo

But you don't have to work out like a professional athlete just to tune up your blood chemistry. Happily, as with many other health benefits of exercise, the effects of exercise on cholesterol metabolism are pretty straightforward: People who spend their lives in a chair or on the couch will have the lowest levels of HDL cholesterol, and those who are most active will have the highest. Even exercise as simple as walking briskly on most days for at least thirty minutes has been shown to significantly increase HDL cholesterol in younger and older women and men.

Exercise Helps Stabilize Blood Pressure

There is now good evidence that light to moderate exercise, performed frequently, can help prevent the rise in blood pressure that the average American experiences with increasing age. There is also evidence that this type of exercise decreases blood pressure in some people with chronic high blood pressure (hypertension). Some of this decrease may result from the weight-reducing effects of exercise, but some of the benefit is due to a "down regulation" of the nervous system. For more information, see the chapter Controlling High Blood Pressure with Exercise.

Exercise Can Help Your State of Mind

Much has been claimed concerning the benefits of exercise on psychological health. Even though many of these claims have been exaggerated—jogging twenty or thirty miles a week will not guarantee eternal bliss—the psychological benefits are still considerable. If you have ever exercised regularly, you are already aware of them. If not, it may be hard to convince you of their existence.

You do not have to exercise to the intensity needed to experience the "runner's high" to reap the psychological benefits—and that is certainly not what we advocate in this book. Moderate exercise will do just fine. For example, regular exercisers report less anxiety and depression and feel they are better able to cope with stress when they exercise than when they don't. Recent research at Stanford has shown that frequent exercise reduces the increases in blood pressure and heart rate caused by stress.

In spite of valiant attempts, researchers have not yet pinned down a cast-iron physiological reason for this improvement in mental state, although some have suggested that the reasons may be found in a reduction of adrenaline in the blood and an increase in the amount of endorphins, a natural tranquilizer produced by the body. However, these biological mechanisms have yet to be substantiated as the cause of improvements in the exerciser's mental state. But we can say, beyond a doubt, that exercise improves mental outlook and the ability to control stress in three ways:

- by providing a socially acceptable way to spend time away from the stresses of everyday life

- by improving self-image, self-esteem, and self-confidence

- by providing a feeling of control over your life

For more on exercise and stress, see the chapter Mind+ Body: The No-Stress Equation.

Self-Test: Do You Think You Could Be in Better Shape?

One way to assess your fitness that requires no equipment is simply to use your intuition. You probably know a lot more about your general condition than you think you do. The best combination of information is a good intuition and quantitative data that backs it up or dispels inaccurate beliefs.

Ask yourself some questions:

1. **How's your stamina?** Regardless of your answer, check it with some facts. Does a dash through the airport leave you winded? Do you go up a staircase quickly, or do you take it step by step, counting every step?

2. **How's your weight?** Are you buying larger and larger sizes every year?

3. **How's your diet?** Do you eat fruits, vegetables, and grains every day?

4. **How's your flexibility?** Do you avoid bending over because you're afraid you may not make it back up?

5. **How many excuses do you have?** Do you feel like you really should exercise more but you just don't have the time, energy, clothes, equipment…?

The self-tests scattered throughout this book will give you more information on specific aspects of your fitness. The chapters in this book will help you tailor an exercise program to your specific needs.

Exercise Helps Slow the Aging Process

Exercise can help to hold back time: It really can make us physiologically younger than our sedentary contemporaries. Researchers who have compared exercisers in their sixties and seventies with sedentary people of the same age have found that exercisers are effectively ten to twenty years younger. Cardiovascular function, body composition, muscle strength and endurance, blood lipids, and appearance are all in significantly

Real Exercise for Real People

The four people you will see demonstrating exercises in this book are all affiliated with the Health Improvement Program of the Stanford Center for Research in Disease Prevention. They are real people, not models—good examples of healthy individuals for their age groups. Tony Thurman is thirty-eight, Terrie Rizzo is forty-nine, Wes Alles is fifty, and Joyce Hanna is sixty-one.

better condition than those of their contemporaries who are growing old in rocking chairs.

We now know that you are never too old to respond to exercise. In fact, older people have the most to gain from exercise: It is essential to maintaining independence and quality of life. And if that isn't enough, you can be sure that the exercisers get more enjoyment out of life!

Exercise Helps Us Live Longer

The human body is designed to take it easy when we are physically active and work harder when we are sedentary: It may seem odd, but when we are physically active, we actually put less wear and tear on our bodies. So it's not surprising that men and women who lead physically active lives live longer on average than those who are sedentary, and suffer less of a disease burden along the way.

For example, in a study of male Harvard University alumni, those who are physically active have a life expectancy three to four years longer than those who are sedentary. This increase in disability-free life expectancy is due to a lower occurrence of chronic degenerative diseases, especially diseases of the cardiovascular system. That is why the American Heart Association has made sedentary lifestyle a major risk factor for heart disease, along with cigarette smoking, high blood pressure, and an abnormal cholesterol profile.

You have nothing to lose, and everything to gain, from adding exercise to your life. And it's never too soon—or too late—to start.

Why Exercise Works

William Haskell, PH.D.

A better understanding of how your body works can't help but translate into an exercise program that is safe and effective.

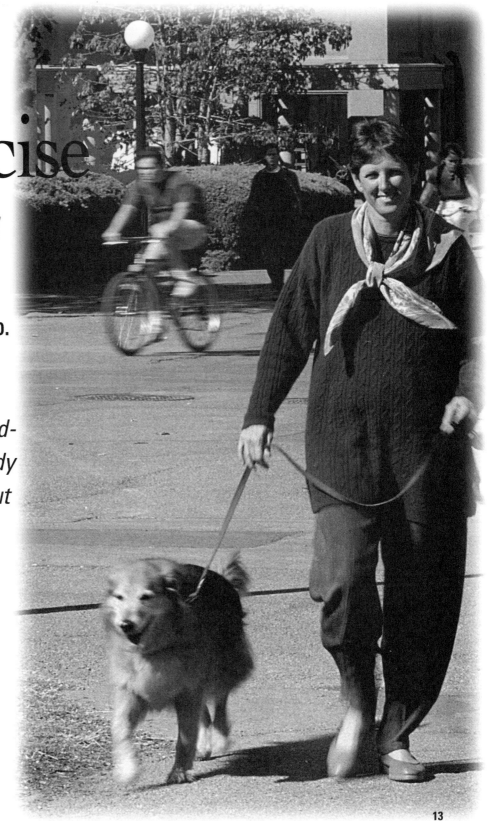

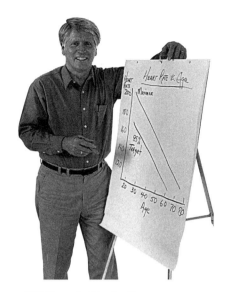

William L. Haskell, PH.D.,
is Professor of Medicine at
Stanford University School of
Medicine, Deputy Director of
Stanford Center for Research in
Disease Prevention, consultant
to the President's Council on
Physical Fitness and Sports, and
past president of the American
College of Sports Medicine. He
participates in a variety of activities, including jogging, hiking,
and skiing.

*D*ESPITE MARK TWAIN'S PRONOUNCEMENT, "The
only exercise I get is being a pallbearer for my
more active friends," writers, philosophers, and scientists have celebrated the benefits of regular exercise for a long time. During the twentieth century, we have
made great strides in understanding what actually happens to
the body during physical activity and also how it contributes
to physical fitness and health.

What Do We Mean by Exercise?

Although we often use the terms physical activity, exercise,
and physical fitness interchangeably, they are actually different
concepts.

Physical activity is any bodily movement produced by the
skeletal muscles, which results in energy expenditure. This
includes any of the countless daily movements we perform
in our occupation, leisure time or sports, conditioning programs, and household activities. We can put these activities
in the following categories:

Exercise (or exercise training) is physical activity that is
planned, structured, and repetitive—such as doing calisthenics, lifting weights, or jogging—performed with the intent of
improving your physical fitness or health.

Physical fitness is a combination of attributes associated
with the development of skills, such as speed and agility, or
with health, such as strength, flexibility, endurance, and body
composition.

So, when we talk about being physically fit, we're really
talking about both health-related fitness and skill-related fit-

ness. If you stick to a well-rounded exercise program, you should see—and feel—improvement in areas of health-related fitness:

- healthy heart and lungs (cardiorespiratory endurance)
- muscular strength
- body composition (fat and lean)
- flexibility

and skill-related fitness:

- agility
- balance
- coordination
- speed
- power
- reaction time

In this chapter, we'll take a look at how physical activity affects our bodies. A better understanding of how your body works can't help but translate into an exercise program that is safe and effective.

How Muscles Gain Strength and Endurance

Muscle strength and endurance are quite separate components of fitness, but they are highly related in many activities.

MUSCLE STRENGTH   When we talk about the strength of a muscle, we're talking about its capacity to exert force through

Myth: **If you are tired at the end of the day, it means that you've had enough exercise.**

Fact: **Not necessarily—lack of exercise can actually make you feel fatigued and worn out.**

contraction of muscle fibers. Since the muscle's force is directly related to its size, people with large muscles have the potential to develop a lot of strength and exert large amounts of force.

Strength is an important fitness component, but not everyone is—or needs to be—equally strong. The optimal amount of strength for each person depends on individual needs and occupations. Fire fighters and construction workers, for example, have strength needs that are quite different from those of a person who works at a desk all day. We can partially explain the differences in strength between individuals and between men and women by such factors as amount of muscle tissue, amount of sex hormones (primarily the male hormone testosterone), and social or cultural influences.

MUSCLE ENDURANCE   Muscle endurance is the ability of any muscle group to repeat muscle contractions against resistance over a period of time. It can also be measured as the amount of time one can sustain a specific muscle contraction. For example, endurance can be measured by the number of times we can successfully maneuver each mogul on the ski slope before becoming tired.

Muscles develop endurance as they develop mechanisms to accommodate the increased demands placed on them. Repeated muscle contractions stimulate an increased blood flow to the muscle, providing the extra oxygen, nutrients, and enzymes necessary for the muscle to continue to work and postpone fatigue.

You can develop your muscle strength and endurance by using *isometric, dynamic,* and *isokinetic* muscle contractions.

While you don't have to understand these concepts in order to get a good workout, it doesn't hurt to know what you're doing!

ISOMETRIC CONTRACTIONS Isometric contractions were popularized by body builder Charles Atlas in the 1950s in his "dynamic tension" program, which promised "ninety-pound weaklings" significant muscular development. Since then, numerous research studies have indicated that strength can be increased with isometric exercises, but not to the extent previously claimed.

Isometric contraction means simply contracting a muscle and holding it for a short period of time without moving— for example, if you were to contract the quadricep muscle of your thigh with the knee extended, and without moving the hip or knee joint. To achieve the best results, maximum contractions must be held for at least six seconds several times per day. The greatest disadvantage of isometrics appears to be that strength is developed only at the angle at which the contraction is held. Thus in order to gain strength through the full range of movement using this technique, a muscle group would have to undergo numerous six-second contractions at various angles in its normal range of movement—and that's quite a bit to ask of the average exerciser.

Older adults or people of any age who have heart disease or high blood pressure should use isometric cautiously. This type of exercise causes an increase in both heart rate and blood pressure. The longer you hold the contraction, the higher they go. This large increase in blood pressure can be dangerous in a person who has heart or artery problems. For more information, see the chapters Exercising After a Heart Attack and Controlling High Blood Pressure with Exercise.

DYNAMIC CONTRACTIONS   A dynamic workout involves moving a weight from one place to another—moving a box from one place to another, or picking up a barbell and putting it down. Isotonic contractions are more universally valuable in developing strength. That is, when force is generated by the muscle, there is movement at the joint.

Effective strength-training programs using dynamic techniques usually apply the principles of *progressive resistance* and *overload*. In the progressive resistance approach, you work with a specific weight, say five pounds, until you can lift it more than ten times (repetitions). To gain strength with the exercise, you add small amounts of weight or resistance, say a pound or two at a time. Thus you progressively increase the resistance. The overload principle says that for improvements in strength to occur, you have to lift heavier weight than you normally do. That is, you overload the muscle relative to what it is usually used to doing. This overload causes the muscle to adapt by increasing its strength.

Greek mythology illustrates both these principles in the story of Milo of Crotona, who set about becoming the strongest man in the world by lifting a young bull each day until the bull was full grown. Any parent who has carried a child every day as it grows from infancy to toddlerhood will understand this principle!

Instead of bulls, dynamic exercisers today can make use of a diverse range of equipment. However, traditional barbells or free weights are still the favorite equipment for serious strength-training aficionados. Novices to weight-training exercise are probably best served by the convenience and safety of facilities that have available a variety of weight-training machines.

Strength development using dynamic contractions is limited by the constant level of resistance throughout the movement. This means that the amount of weight you lift is limited to the maximum that can be lifted at the weakest point in the muscle group's range of contraction.

ISOKINETIC CONTRACTIONS Isokinetic contractions attempt to address the limitations of strength development associated with both dynamic and isometric contractions. In an isokinetic contraction, the speed of the contraction remains constant, but the resistance offered by the machine matches the individual's capability throughout the range of motion. This effect, called *accommodating resistance*, permits a maximum contraction to be performed through a full range of movement.

The isokinetic contraction was first introduced in 1968 by a bioengineer, James Perrine, who developed a speed-controlled dynamometer called a Cybex machine. Many other devices have now been developed that provide a similar type of variable resistance. The cost of this type of equipment is usually more than individuals can afford on their own, and these machines are usually found in health clubs and rehabilitation settings.

You can use dynamic or isokinetic equipment to develop both muscle strength and endurance. However, exercise programs that are designed to develop strength or endurance vary in the relationship between the amount of resistance and

Myth: If your heart and lungs are in good shape, that means you're physically fit.

Fact: Fitness actually has four components: cardiorespiratory endurance, flexibility, muscular strength, and body composition.

"This book presents up-to-the minute information in exercise science. The SCDRP is internationally recognized for research in health promotion." —**Terrie Rizzo**

number of repetitions. If strength is the main requirement, the number of repetitions for an exercise is kept low and the resistance is high. In a muscular endurance program, the repetitions are high and the resistance is low. For more detailed information, see the chapter Using Your Muscles for Life.

How We Build Cardiovascular Endurance

Cardiovascular endurance—the ability of the heart to effectively pump blood to the working muscles—is referred to by various names, including stamina, aerobic fitness, aerobic capacity, and functional capacity. The term *aerobic fitness* is usually used to describe cardiovascular endurance, but *functional capacity* or *maximal oxygen consumption (VO₂max)* are the more accepted scientific terms.

Your ability to exercise continuously for short or long periods of time depends on how effectively your heart, lungs, arteries, capillaries, cells, and veins can transfer oxygen, carbon dioxide, nutrients, and waste products to and from the working muscles. As soon as you start to exercise, your body adapts to the increased energy demands being placed on it. Energy stores of glycogen are mobilized within the muscles to provide the fuel necessary for them to contract. At the same time, since the muscles also need more oxygen, the heart and respiration rates increase to provide more oxygenated blood.

As long as your working muscles can receive an adequate amount of oxygen to continue a process called oxidation in the muscle cells, exercise can continue and you don't feel fatigue. This type of exercise is frequently referred to as *aerobic exercise.* When your muscles work at a rate that outstrips the supply of oxygen delivered to them, waste products such as lactic acid build up in them and causes fatigue. This is called *anaerobic exercise* (exercise without oxygen), and fatigue results in a short period of time.

VO$_2$MAX   Oxygen supply for the muscles depends on a healthy heart, which must make more oxygen available to the muscles by increasing its rate of contraction and the amount of blood pumped per beat (stroke volume). As heart rate and stroke volume increase, more blood circulates each minute, thereby increasing the cardiac output of the heart.

As the cardiac output is increased, more oxygen is made available to the working muscle. The maximum amount of oxygen that a person can deliver to the body is called their maximum oxygen uptake, or aerobic capacity (VO$_2$max).

Further, since a person's maximal oxygen uptake depends on an efficient respiratory system, measurement of maximal oxygen uptake is one of the very best measurements of dynamic heart and lung function.

Age, sex, genetics, and lifestyle contribute to a wide variation among the population regarding this fitness measure. People who lead active lifestyles, whatever their age, have higher VO$_2$max levels than their sedentary counterparts.

THE FITT PRINCIPLE   Cardiovascular endurance can be developed by a training program based on variations of the FITT principle: that is, with the *frequency, intensity, time*, and *type of exercise* necessary to produce physiological changes over weeks or months. These may include favorable changes in:

Myth: Exercise is boring.

Fact: Doing the same thing over and over again is boring! Varying your exercise activities helps prevent boredom and repetition and helps balance conditioning.

- resting heart rate and blood pressure, submaximal exercise heart rate, and blood pressure and body weight
- body composition (the percentages of the body that are muscle and bone by comparison with body fat)
- lipoproteins (chemical structures present in the blood that carry fat, proteins, and cholesterol)
- fat and carbohydrate metabolism (the way the body uses fat and sugar carried in the blood)
- bone mineralization

Accompanying psychological changes may include less stress, depression, and anxiety, and improvement in self-image.

The training intensity necessary to produce such physiological and psychological change varies from one person to another and is different for people of different ages, sexes, and health status. However, if you select the appropriate type of exercise for your current level of fitness and set it at the proper intensity, duration, and frequency, then you should see improvements in physical fitness and associated health benefits.

Your exercise program should follow three basic principles of exercise training:

- *overload* (doing more than was done previously)
- *specificity* (relating the activity to your specific needs)
- *progression* (starting out slowly and adding small increments of time, intensity, and/or distance as fitness improves).

For more information, see the chapter Creating Your Own Exercise Program.

A Physical Activity Plan for Every Age

Every age group has its own needs when it comes to a physical activity plan. Where do your needs fit in?

Major Health-Fitness Goals	**Physical Activity Plan**
YOUTH (1 TO 14 YEARS)	
• Optimal physical growth and development • Good psychological adjustment • Develop interest and skills for active lifestyle as adult • Reduction of coronary heart disease risk factors	**T:** Emphasis on large muscle, dynamic exercise; moving body over distance and against gravity; some heavy resistive activity and flexibility exercise **I:** Moderate to vigorous intensity **D:** Total of more than 30 minutes per day in one or more sessions **F:** Every day **G:** Increased activity to and from school
MOST YOUNG ADULTS (15 TO 24 YEARS)	
• Optimal physical growth and development • Good psychological adjustment • Develop interest and skills for active lifestyle as adult • Reduction of coronary heart disease risk factors	**T:** Emphasis on large muscle, dynamic strength, and flexibility exercise **I:** Moderate to vigorous intensity (more than 50 percent VO_2max) **D:** Total of more than 30 minutes per session (more than 4 kilocalories per kilogram of body weight) **F:** At least every other day **G:** Increased activity to and from school
ADULTS (25 TO 65 YEARS)	
• Prevention and treatment of coronary heart disease • Prevention and treatment of Type II diabetes • Maintenance of optimal body composition • Enhance psychological status • Retain musculoskeletal integrity	**T:** Emphasis on large muscle dynamic exercise; some heavy resistive and flexibility exercises **I:** Moderate intensity (more than 50 percent VO_2max) **D:** Total of more than 30 minutes per session (more than 4 kilocalories per kilogram of body weight) **F:** At least every other day **G:** Lower-level activities (e.g., walking) every day
OLDER ADULTS (OVER 65 YEARS)	
• Maintain general functional capacity • Retain musculoskeletal integrity and balance • Enhance psychological status • Prevent and treat coronary heart disease and Type II diabetes	**T:** Emphasis on moving about, flexibility, and some resistive exercises **I:** Moderate intensity (overload with slow progression) **D:** Based on capacity of individual, up to 60 minutes per day in multiple sessions **F:** Every day **G:** Lower-level activities (e.g., walking) every day

T = Type of Exercise
I = Intensity
D = Duration or amount
F = Frequency of exercise session
G = Goal

Source: *Public Health Report* (April 1985).

CARDIOVASCULAR WORKOUTS A variety of training programs can develop cardiovascular endurance. Essentially, they consist of or combine the following methods:

- *interval training* (exercise and rest intervals are organized in various combinations)

- *continuous training* (exercise intensity is adjusted to permit long bouts of continuous exercise)

- *interval-circuit training* (running, walking, and calisthenic exercise are incorporated into a circuit that can vary in distance and time).

Flexibility

Many people become aware of flexibility—the range of movement of limbs around a joint—only as they get older, or if they participate in activities where its presence or absence clearly affects their physical performance. Following recovery from an injury such as a fractured limb, lack of flexibility becomes quite apparent.

When you break your arm and it is set in a cast, you don't use the muscles and the joint for a number of weeks. With disuse, the muscle atrophies, or grows smaller. Not only are muscle size and strength reduced considerably, range of movement of the limb is also severely compromised. When the cast is removed, you can't use your arm nearly as well as you could before the break, and you need a program of rehabilitation exercises to help it resume its previous function. Strength and flexibility exercises are an important part of this rehabilitation process.

Myth: For quick energy, you should eat foods high in sugar before exercising.

Fact: It takes twenty to thirty minutes for the energy from sugar to become available to your muscles.

Flexibility varies among different joints in the body, depending on the structure and the function of the joint. The shoulder and knee joints, for example, are structurally very different. The shoulder joint has a much greater range of motion than the knee. The range of motion of a joint is influenced by structures that surround it, such as muscle, ligaments, and tendons. In order to prevent injury, it is important to establish an appropriate balance between strength and flexibility. Excessive range of motion in a joint or an imbalance in strength of muscles surrounding a joint can increase risk of an injury.

FLEXIBILITY EXERCISES   Flexibility exercises increase the range of motion of a joint, allowing muscles to exert strength (force) for a longer period of time. This is particularly noticeable in activities like swimming, gymnastics, and golf, where increased flexibility in the wrist, elbow, and shoulder joints can enhance performance. Also, people who have adequate flexibility are less likely to incur injuries.

In the past, flexibility exercises were recommended as part of the warm-up period that precedes exercise. Today, however, we have found that some light form of aerobic activity such as walking or slow jogging is important to sufficiently warm up the musculoskeletal system. The increased body temperature increases the blood supply, and thus prepares both muscles and joints for efficient stretching and activity.

The wide variety of flexibility exercises that have been developed fit into one of four categories: static, ballistic, dynamic, and PNF stretches.

Static stretches. In static stretching, the body part being exercised is stretched lightly to lengthen the muscle and tendons, and the stretched position is then held for a period of twenty to thirty seconds. Slow breathing can enhance relaxation during this stretch. During the period of stretch, the length of the muscle will slowly increase, thus ensuring an optimal length over which the muscle will be able to contract during subsequent exercise. This method is the safest, most practical, and most effective for most people.

Ballistic stretches. Ballistic stretches involve visible movement. The typical ballistic stretch uses the momentum of body weight to induce the stretch. This form of "bouncy" or "jerky" stretching is not recommended: It can compromise certain reflex mechanisms in the muscles and tendons surrounding the joint and may result in injury.

Dynamic stretches. Dynamic stretches, which incorporate slow movements, have been used for many years by dancers and those who practice yoga. The dynamic stretch is done in a slow and controlled manner throughout the range of movement of the specific activity to he performed. Since the stretch is controlled, there is a minimal risk of injury to the muscle or joint.

PNF stretches. A more recent approach to flexibility exercise is called *proprioceptive neuromuscular facilitation* (PNF). In this method of muscle and joint stretching, the muscle is first tightened (contracted) and then statically stretched. Although flexibility can be achieved by this method, residual muscle soreness has also been reported. This method also requires a partner and is more time-consuming to perform than the other methods. See the chapter Stretching for Flexibility to learn more.

Body Composition

When we talk about body composition in relation to health and exercise, we mean the proportion of the body that is fat weight and the proportion that is lean, muscle weight. The only accurate way to measure body composition directly is to dissect the body and literally weigh each of its various tissue components—not very practical for those interested in participating in exercise after the assessment has been completed! Fortunately, there are a few other assessment techniques.

MEASURING BODY COMPOSITION Two popular techniques that have been used in the past to estimate body composition include skin-fold and girth measurements. Recent technological advances have resulted in some attempts to use magnetic resonance imaging (MRI) and bioelectrical impedance.

The most widely used and accurate indirect assessment method to determine body composition is *hydrostatic weighing*. This method determines body density (body density = body weight/body volume) by weighing a person on an accurate scale in air, then weighing the person submerged in water after he or she has expired as much air as possible from the lungs. After corrections and calculations are made to this information, the result is a determination of the person's lean body weight and fat weight as a percentage of total body weight.

IDEAL BODY COMPOSITION What is the ideal body weight and composition that is associated with optimal health, and how can we achieve it? Research suggests that for men the ideal amount of body fat is between 15 percent and 18 percent of total body weight, and for women body fat should be

How Many Calories Can I Burn in Cardiovascular Exercise?

The following are some of the better cardiovascular-respiratory exercises and the number of kcal expended per hour of the exercise. Select several activities that are enjoyable, and use them in such a way that you look forward to your scheduled exercise sessions rather than dread them.

Activity	kcal per hour*	Activity	kcal per hour*
Badminton, competitive singles	480	Skiing, downhill, vigorous	600
Basketball	360–660	Skiing, cross-country	
Bicycling		2.5 mph	560
10 mph	420	4 mph	600
11 mph	480	8 mph	1,020
12 mph	600	Swimming,	
Calisthenics, heavy	600	25-50 yards per minute	360–750
Handball, competitive	660	Walking	
Rope skipping, vigorous	800	level road, 4 mph	420
Rowing machine	840	upstairs	600–1,080
Running		uphill, 3.5 mph	480–900
5 mph	600	Gardening,	
6 mph	750	much lifting, stooping, digging	500
7 mph	870	Mowing, pushing hand mower	450
8 mph	1,020	Sawing hardwood	600
9 mph	1,130	Shoveling, heavy	660
Skating, ice or inline, rapid	700	Wood chopping	560

*Caloric consumption is based on a 150-pound person. There is a 10 percent increase in caloric consumption for each 15 pounds over this weight, and a 10 percent decrease for each 15 pounds under.

Source: E. L. Wynder, *The Book of Health, The American Health Foundation* (New York: Franklin Watts, 1981.) Used with permission.

between 22 percent and 25 percent of total body weight. However, it is important to remember that individual variation other than sex, such as age and physical activity level, can result in changes in these percentages.

Although body build (the genetic contribution to our form and structure) and body size (height and mass) can only be changed minimally by a regular exercise program, significant change can occur in body composition. For example, as most people get older they experience a decrease in muscle mass and an increase in body fat and total body weight. Although this is the norm for the majority of the American population, substantial evidence indicates these changes are not inevitable.

People who maintain an active lifestyle that includes regular physical activity using the large muscle groups in the body are able to maintain optimal body weight and body composition. Regular exercise increases lean body weight and decreases fat weight. This is doubly desirable because muscle mass is more active metabolically than fat—that is, it has greater energy needs than fat (which is primarily a storage facility for energy). Increasing muscle mass is like increasing engine capacity. With a larger engine, we use more fuel, and since most of the fuel is stored in fat, we are able to effectively reduce our fat stores and favorably affect our body composition.

Effective weight and body composition control involves both caloric expenditure (exercise) as well as caloric restriction (diet). The relative merits of both methods of controlling body weight and composition have received substantial research attention in the past (see the chapter Eat Well, Be Well for more information). In 1985, a National Institutes of Health consensus panel on obesity underscored the importance of optimal body composition by agreeing that losing weight is not just a matter of vanity, it is a matter of health.

Understanding Your Body

Physical fitness is important to the development of good health. It helps us avoid the significant negative physiological and psychological effects on health that results from inactivity and deconditioning.

Muscular strength and endurance, cardiovascular endurance, flexibility, and body composition all have an impact on physical fitness and health. Understanding the effects of exercise and physical activity on each of these is important if we are to experience the health benefits of exercise and avoid the health risks.

Eat Well, Be Well

Marcia L. Stefanick, PH.D.

Researchers agree that the combination of exercise and a lower-calorie diet results in much greater weight loss than diet alone.

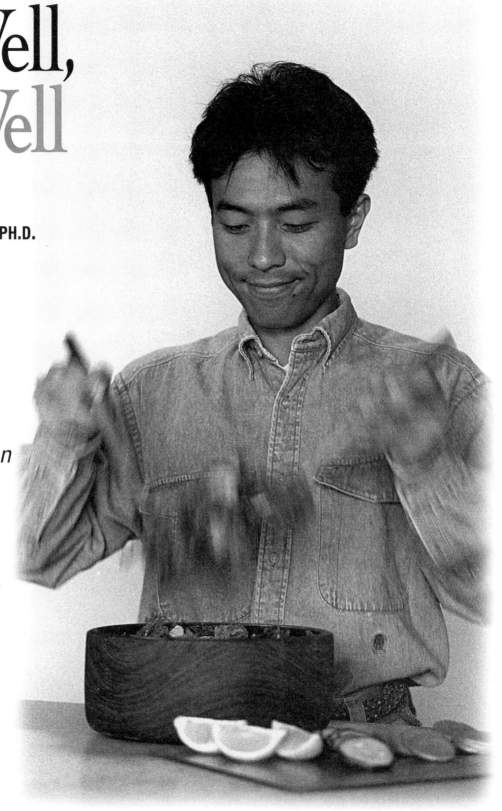

YEAR BY YEAR, MOST OF US are growing fatter. Fifteen years ago, one-fourth of adult Americans were overweight. Today, according to the most recent National Health and Nutrition Examination Survey, this number has leaped to one-third. Women in general seem to be particularly prone to weight gain—they are twice as likely to gain more than ten pounds over a ten-year period than men.

This is not welcome news. Research shows that being overweight directly affects health—and the effect is not a good one. Obesity is related to several major chronic diseases: heart disease (the leading cause of disease and death in men and women in this country); several major cancers (including colorectal cancer, prostate cancer, breast, uterine, and ovarian cancers); chronic high blood pressure (hypertension); diabetes; and unfavorable cholesterol levels, particularly low levels of HDL, the "good cholesterol," and high levels of fats in the blood (triglycerides). Gallbladder disease is also six times more prevalent in overweight people. Clearly, the high incidence of obesity in the United States poses a serious public health concern.

Why We Gain Weight

Most researchers agree that we gain weight when our energy (caloric) intake chronically exceeds our energy expenditure. In other words, if we eat more calories than our bodies burn, we will gain weight (fat).

For most people, the solution is: Eat less and exercise more, and do it consistently. The Council of Scientific Affairs of the American Medical Association cited the three essential

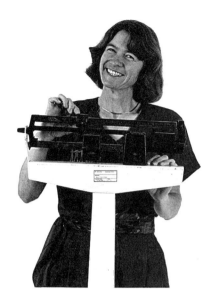

Marcia L. Stefanick, PH.D., is Senior Research Scientist at the Stanford Center for Research in Disease Prevention. She is Principal Investigator for the NIH Women's Health Initiative (WHI) and Post-Menopausal Estrogen/Progestin Interventions (PEPI); Co-Principal Investigator and Project Director for the Diet and Exercise for Elevated (Cardiovascular) Risk Trial (DEER). She was also Co-Principal Investigator for the Heart and Estrogen Replacement Study (HERS). Her primary form of aerobic exercise is running.

Yo-Yo Dieting: Why We Lose and Gain and Lose and Gain

Most people who diet do so over and over and over, losing and gaining the same ten or twenty pounds again and again. If you are one of these people, you may have given up hope long ago. But take heart: There is a way to stop the yo-yo diet effect.

When we lose weight through exercise, most of the weight we lose is fat. When we lose weight through dieting, without exercise, we lose fat but we also lose a considerable amount of lean body mass, including muscle mass. This results in a decrease in basal or resting metabolic rate—that is, our body slows down in its ability to burn calories. This means that to maintain the lower weight, we must further reduce caloric intake; otherwise, weight regain is almost inevitable, most of it fat weight. This, in turn, means that the resting metabolic rate is reduced at the former weight, so we must "diet" just to prevent further weight gain rather than to lose weight. The result is what is popularly called "yo-yo" dieting—losing, gaining, losing, gaining, in a seemingly endless cycle. Fortunately, exercise offers a real and lasting way out.

components of a weight-control program as diet, exercise, and behavior modification. Most Americans, however, don't follow this plan.

National surveys tell us that among people who are trying to lose weight, about 64 percent of the women and 44 percent of the men do it solely by cutting calories; half as many of each try to lose weight solely by increasing their levels of physical activity. Only 31 percent of overweight women and 20 percent of overweight men eat less and exercise more. This is a shame, because researchers agree that the combination of exercise and a lower-calorie diet results in much greater weight loss than diet alone. Furthermore, exercise is one of the few factors that is clearly associated with successful long-term weight maintenance.

Lose Fat, Not Muscle

The goal of every weight-loss program should be *fat* weight loss, not total weight loss. The key is patience: You can't lose fat overnight.

It takes longer to lose fat weight than you may be used to on total weight loss diets. On these diets, we quickly lose water and stored carbohydrate or protein. Not surprisingly, such rapid losses are also quickly reversed, so that a person who loses ten pounds in a week or two by seriously cutting calories is likely to gain it all back in an equally short period.

Similarly, just starting an exercise program does not guarantee weight loss, particularly at the outset. At the beginning, you must expend between 3,000 and 3,500 calories, relative to caloric intake, to lose one pound—enough energy to support about thirty miles of walking or running.

OBSTACLES   At the beginning of any exercise and diet program, you will encounter some confounding—but not insurmountable—obstacles.

Hunger. Hunger can be a problem. Some people experience an increase in appetite when they begin an exercise program, leading them to eat enough calories to equal or exceed the amount of increased energy expenditure possible at the outset of the program, thereby precluding weight loss.

Fatigue. Fatigue is another problem. Some people, particularly if they are quite unfit initially, do less outside their exercise program and sleep more because of exercise-induced fatigue. This means that even though they feel like they are working hard, the amount of energy they are expending is

Myth: Exercise makes you hungrier, so you end up eating more.

Fact: Moderate exercise diminishes appetite. But even if you do eat more as a result of exercise, you burn more calories—so you can eat more and weigh less!

unchanged or even reduced over the course of a twenty-four-hour period.

Weight increase. People who have done virtually no previous exercise may have a slight increase in lean weight when they initiate an exercise program because they are building muscle. They are also gaining some water weight to accommodate water loss during sweating. These gains may equal or exceed fat weight losses, again resulting in no change or even an increase in total weight during the initial weeks of the program.

DON'T GIVE UP! If you are eager to lose a lot of weight in a short period, all of this may sound very discouraging. But don't give up! Regular exercise causes our bodies to change in ways that help us burn more fat during exercise. These changes, combined with simple modifications in diet, can offset problems associated with increased appetite. Other physiological adaptations to exercise not only reduce fatigue and enable you to feel more energetic in general, they increase energy expenditure during exercise.

Finally, you will not continue to gain lean weight unless you are engaged in body building or other heavy resistance exercise. Water-weight gain also does not continue to increase, so fat weight loss become more obvious as time goes on. Although this adaptation process may take two to three months, the weight will begin to come off very easily. If you continue to exercise, as little as one mile of walking a day (roughly fifteen or twenty minutes of effort) will bring about ten pounds of fat weight loss over the course of a year with little, if any, loss of lean body mass. Patience pays off.

Myth: Being overweight makes exercising dangerous.

Fact: The primary risk is trying to accomplish your goals in a hurry by exercising too much and too quickly. When you follow recommended guidelines, exercise is a good way to help you manage your weight.

How Aerobic Exercise Burns Fat

From the moment we start to do physical activity, our muscles need more and more fuel. And the fuel they want for prolonged low- to moderate-intensity exercise is fat. Only at high-intensity work is glycogen (the fuel source in carbohydrates) the predominant energy source. Glycogen, however, is quickly depleted, and exercise must stop or intensity must be reduced. At this point fat again becomes the predominant fuel.

This does not mean that we should eat more fat! Even people of average weight have plenty of fat on board to get through most exercise bouts, and burning fat instead of carbohydrates means slow going. Fortunately, after two or three months of steady exercise, we have an even greater ability to use fat as fuel during light or moderate exercise without depleting glycogen. So we can go further slightly faster, without getting tired.

Aerobic exercise stimulates the release of fat from fat tissues so it can be burned by the working muscle. In addition to changes in the muscle cells that enhance their ability to burn more fat (and spare glycogen, for that "kick" at the end), there are many adaptations in fat cells, and the hormone systems that regulate them, that further enhance reduction of body fat with exercise training.

FAT AS FUEL   The only fats that serve as important metabolic fuels are free fatty acids (FFA) and their storage form, triglycerides, which are stored primarily in adipose tissue—that is, fat. *Lipolysis*, the release of fats from adipose tissue, is stimulated by two hormones—norepinephrine (NE) and epi-

> *"Most people can't maintain weight loss simply by cutting calories. Exercise is essential to healthy weight control, and it becomes more important with age."* —**Terrie Rizzo**

nephrine (EPI), which are released by the part of the nervous system that controls the stress responses—fright, fight, and flight. As blood flow increases to the exercising muscle, the FFA released from adipose tissue is carried to the muscle; however, fat metabolism can only be used in the presence of oxygen—that is, aerobically.

MUSCLES AND FAT   There are two basic types of muscle fibers: slow-twitch, oxidative (often called "red") and fast-twitch, glycolytic (often called "white"). The *red muscle fibers* are responsible for most burning of FFA.

Red muscle fibers specialize in aerobic metabolism. They get their "red" appearance from the rich blood supply that provides them with FFA and oxygen, and they contain myoglobin, a protein similar to hemoglobin in its ability to bind oxygen.

In contrast, *white muscle fibers* utilize glycogen almost exclusively and have little ability to burn fat. Red muscle fibers are mainly activated during exercise of moderate intensity, while white fibers are activated during high-intensity exercise.

Each person is born with a different amount of red and white fibers—some have more white than red, some more red than white. The relative amounts contribute to our ability to metabolize fat, determining whether we will be more able to perform endurance-type sports (which require mostly red fibers) or speed and power-type sports (which require mostly white fibers).

This does not mean that an endurance athlete must be slow, as is clearly demonstrated by Olympic marathoners, cyclists, and distance swimmers (who have 85 percent red fibers in their thigh muscles compared to Olympic sprinters, who have 85 percent white fibers): White fibers can become endurance trained and evolve into fast-twitch, oxidative (often called "pink") fibers. Nonetheless, a "born" marathoner can never be as fast as a "born" sprinter, at a short distance.

Apples and Pears: Men and Women and Fat

Many people believe that women have more trouble losing weight, particularly through exercise, than men do. Whether this is true remains unclear; however, women generally deposit fat differently than men do.

Women tend to have more subcutaneous fat—fat deposited under the skin—particularly at certain sites, such as the upper arms, thighs, buttocks, and breasts. Men are more likely to have fat in the midsection and abdominal region, commonly called "beer-belly" fat. A large amount of the male-type fat is located within the abdominal cavity, in large pads around the internal organs, and is generally referred to as "visceral" fat.

These patterns are so common that they are referred to as female-type and male-type. Because the female type is generally associated with a smaller waist and larger hips, it is often called a "pear" shape; while the male type, with larger waist and smaller hips, is often called an "apple" shape.

WHY APPLES MAY LOSE WEIGHT FASTER   One possible explanation for the problems associated with visceral fat is that FFA released from these spots are more likely to hit the

Myth: Exercise reduces cholesterol.

Fact: Exercise alone may increase the level of "good" cholesterol, but the best way to lower total cholesterol is the combination of diet and exercise.

Apples and Pears: What's Your WHR?

The ratio of waist circumference (at the narrowest spot) to hip girth (at the widest spot) is called the waist-to-hip ratio, or WHR. Because a large WHR (apple shape) has been shown to be associated with a greater incidence of most obesity-related disorders—including heart disease, high blood pressure, diabetes, low HDL-cholesterol, high triglycerides, gallbladder disease, and several major cancers—it is recommended that women have a WHR equal to or less than 0.80, and that men have a WHR equal to or less than 0.90.

To find your WHR, divide your waist measurement by your hip measurement. For example if your waist measures 28 inches and your hips measure 38 inches, your WHR is: 28 ÷ 38 = 0.73

liver in high concentration than FFA released from other sites. This in turn affects cholesterol metabolism (promoting reduced HDL-cholesterol) and triglyceride production (promoting increased triglyceride levels, which then promotes diabetes), as well as other liver functions, which lead to the other harmful physiological effects.

The sympathetic nervous system controls the release of FFA at the time of exercise. Interestingly, NE and EPI have been shown to be more able to bring about fat release from visceral fat cells than from subcutaneous fat cells. What's more, certain subcutaneous fat depots are more responsive to these sympathetic hormones than others—for example, waist-area subcutaneous fat is more likely to be released than thigh or buttocks fat.

These fat depots also differ in how they respond to insulin, which works to prevent fat release (thereby favoring fat storage). Thigh and buttocks fat is very responsive to insulin, while visceral fat is much less so. Together, these differences favor release of fat from the "male" storage sites and inhibit release from the "female" sites with exercise. Presumably, this could lead to greater fat loss in apples than pears during exercise. (On the downside, stress also promotes release of fat from these sites. This may cause all the problems associated with a high WHR if muscles are not active to put the released fat to good use as fuel.)

The Fats of Life

Did you ever wonder where those hidden fat calories are coming from? In this typical fast-food meal, 41 percent of the calories are from fat!

FOOD ITEM	CALORIES	FAT (GRAMS)	PROTEIN (GRAMS)
Fast-food burger	563	33	24.5
Large French fries	350	17	4.5
Chocolate shake	383	9	10
Total	1,296	59	39

While it is true that many more women are pear-shaped than men, it is also true that many women are more apple shaped than pear shaped. If it is true that apples lose weight with exercise more easily than pears (which remains to be proven), a large number of women would find exercise-induced weight loss to be quite effective. And since most obesity-related health complications are associated with the high WHR, it is these women (and men!) who will benefit the most by exercise.

Eat Your Fruits and Vegetables

How do the types of foods we eat affect weight gain? Many investigators have suggested that eating fats may contribute more to obesity than eating equal calories from other food sources. Several studies have failed to show a strong relationship between caloric intake and fatness, although it is very difficult to accurately assess what people actually eat. However, the percent of calories from fat, particularly saturated fat intake, has been repeatedly shown to relate to obesity.

Because fat provides such high calories, it is easy to consume a lot of calories with relatively little food. Consequently, changing the diet to one high in complex carbohydrates (grains, fruits, and vegetables) as opposed to simple sugars gives some people the feeling that they must eat an inordinate amount to satisfy hunger, and eating such large volumes of food may seem counterproductive to the person eager to lose

Burning It Up

Here's the exercise it takes to burn the fast-food meal of 1,296 calories.

ACTIVITY	DURATION
Swimming @ 600 calories/hour	2.2 hours
Jogging @ 500 calories/hour	2.3 hours
Dancing @ 384 calories/hour	3.4 hours
Golf @ more than 200 calories/hour	10.8 hours

weight. If you want to maintain or lose weight and control hunger, you should eat foods that are low in fat and simple sugars, but high in complex carbohydrates and high in fiber.

A high-fat diet is also a very bad idea for a successful exercise program. Many studies have shown that diets high in fat are associated with early fatigue during exercise, especially if one tries to increase speed; this in turn limits the amount of exercise one performs, which reduces the amount of fat that will be burned. The best dietary advice for exercise is to consume a low-fat diet (25 to 30 percent of calories from fat) that is high in carbohydrates (55 to 60 percent), with the rest consisting of protein (15 percent).

There is no evidence that one must consume a high-protein diet to increase muscle strength, even with body-building exercises. In fact, excess protein will be converted to fat. (If you are diabetic or have another metabolic disorder, you may need to follow different fat and carbohydrate guidelines. Consult your physician or a clinical dietitian.)

Diet + Exercise = Weight Loss

It is important to eat enough calories to keep your energy levels up; but if you wish to lose weight, it is reasonable to combine caloric reduction (of about 500 calories per day) with exercise to achieve the best possible weight loss. The object of a diet- and exercise-based weight-loss program should be to minimize the diet-induced loss of lean weight, while maximizing the loss of fat weight by the combination of caloric restriction (particularly fat calories) with aerobic (endurance) exercise. Addition of resistance ("weight") training is likely to facilitate protection of lean body weight.

We still have a lot to learn about the optimal diet and exercise program for weight loss and athletic performance. Among other parameters, the effectiveness of exercise on weight loss may be influenced by the following:

- the type (endurance, resistance, anaerobic), intensity or speed, frequency, and length of each session of exercise, and the duration of the training program

- where the fat is located and the nature of the excess fat

- the composition and caloric content of the diet

Finally, even if you have been very successful at weight loss in an intensive program, you must eventually figure things out for yourself. How are you going to eat real food and maintain an activity level that promotes weight maintenance for the rest of your life?

A sedentary person who adopts an exercise program will more than likely improve his or her health, even if there is no weight loss. This may be particularly important for a woman with female-pattern obesity to realize, because she may have more trouble losing weight than men and women with the male fat pattern.

Although few studies have systematically researched the effects of weight loss on women's health, even modest weight loss—a 5 percent reduction in body weight—seems to yield significant long-term improvements in high blood pressure, unhealthy cholesterol and triglyceride profiles, diabetes, and

What Should I Eat?

To lose or maintain your weight and control hunger: Eat foods that are low in fat, high in complex carbohydrates, and with a high fiber content. For example:

- fresh fruits

- fresh vegetables

- whole grains (brown rice, bulgar wheat, wild rice)

- whole-grain breads

- pasta

To maintain a successful exercise program: Eat a low-fat diet (get 25 to 30 percent of your calories from fat) that is high in complex carbohydrates (55 to 60 percent), and the rest consisting of protein (15 percent).

Snacks That Are Good for You

Breads and Crackers (with no added fat):
- whole-grain bread
- bagels
- English muffins
- French bread
- pita bread
- tortillas
- breadsticks
- rice cakes
- Armenian cracker bread
- melba toast
- matzo
- pretzels, unsalted
- rye crackers
- popcorn, air-popped

Fruits and Vegetables:
- fresh fruit
- fresh vegetables
- canned fruit, packed in its own juice
- dried fruit
- unsweetened applesauce

Sweets:
- fig bars
- ginger snaps
- Graham crackers
- nonfat cookies
- low-fat banana bread
- sorbet
- nonfat frozen yogurt
- frozen tofu dessert
- fruit-juice popsicle

Drinks:
- yogurt-and-fruit blended smoothie
- nonfat milk mixed with cocoa powder
- fruit juice

Cereals:
- shredded wheat
- puffed wheat, corn, rice
- naturally sweetened whole grain cereals

Other:
- low-fat, low-sodium canned soups
- low-sodium canned beans
- baked potatoes
- nonfat or low-fat yogurt, fruit or plain
- raw, unsalted nuts
- part-skim or nonfat mozzarella cheese
- nonfat cottage cheese
- low-fat ricotta cheese
- tuna packed in water

heart disease. Independent of weight loss, there is mounting evidence that the combination of adequate calcium intake and weight-bearing exercise reduces osteoporosis.

The evidence for benefits of exercise, with or without weight loss, is even stronger in men, on whom more studies have been conducted. Therefore both men and women should trust the health benefits of taking up an exercise program for weight loss: You'll not only feel better, you'll give yourself a jump start on losing fat and keeping it off.

Mind + Body: The *No-Stress* Equation

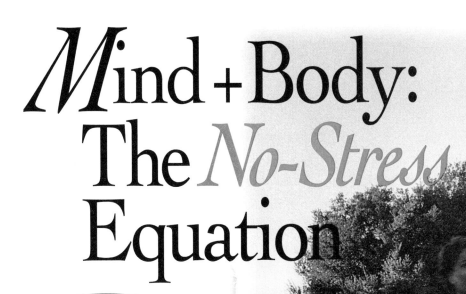

Abby King, PH.D.
C. Barr Taylor, M.D.
Kenneth R. Pelletier, PH.D.

Too much stress can make you more vulnerable to disease and disability. A combination of exercise and relaxation techniques can help you dissolve stress and be more peaceful.

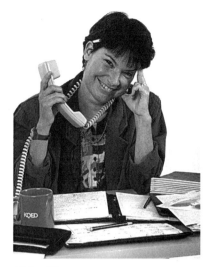

Abby King, PH.D., is Assistant Professor of Health Research and Policy and Medicine, Stanford University School of Medicine, and Senior Research Scientist, SCDRP. She likes to hike, dance, walk, use the stair-stepper, and jog.

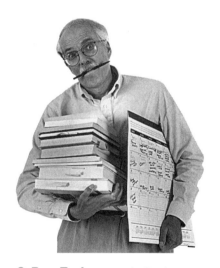

C. Barr Taylor, M.D., is Professor of Psychiatry at Stanford Medical School, Co-Director of the Stanford Cardiac Rehabilitation Program, and Director of Behavioral Science for the Stanford Heart Disease Prevention Program.

*I*N ONE WAY OR ANOTHER, stress contributes to most physical or emotional disorders. It may initiate some problems like skin eruptions or exacerbate others like high blood pressure. And emotionally, sustained stress is associated with anxiety and depression. It interferes with our ability to concentrate, to make decisions, to relax, and to get along with our colleagues and family.

We don't know exactly how stress plays a part in these problems. We do know, however, that there are multiple facets of stress, including positive ones.

Think about the last wedding you participated in or the last vacation you embarked on. While joyous occasions, they no doubt involved some stress—who hasn't remarked upon their return that "I need a vacation to recuperate from my vacation"? Positive stress can excite us to new levels of creativity and energy. It is termed "eustress" to distinguish it from "distress." It's the latter, when it's unremitting, chronic, or uncontrollable, that becomes dangerous.

Where Stress Comes From, Where It Goes

Left over in our bodies from prehistoric days is the "flight-or-fight" response to the threat of perceived threats and demands. Its presence allowed us to either escape or eventually conquer threats of mastodons and saber-toothed tigers. Today, it's not so easy to fight or flee employers, rebellious children, and surly civil servants.

Instead, we live with the anxiety they create, and our bodies respond by getting ready for battles that never take place.

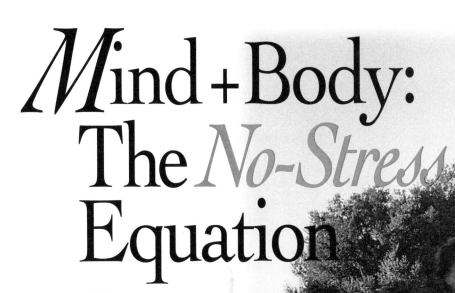

Repeated, chronic activation of your flight-or-fight response can make you more vulnerable to disease and disability.

Moreover, if you use caffeine, tobacco, or alcohol to try to reduce stress, your health may be further endangered. Even resorting to consumption of convenient, high-fat, fast foods —because you're too revved up to slow down and prepare a well-balanced meal—may tend to damage your health in the long run.

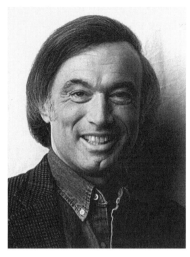

Kenneth R. Pelletier, PH.D., is Clinical Associate Professor of Medicine in the Department of Medicine, and Director of the Stanford Corporate Health Program, a collaborative program between Stanford and twenty major corporations. He is the author of seven major books, including the international bestseller *Mind as Healer, Mind as Slayer.* His program of exercise includes swimming, horseback riding, and jogging, and his favorite sport, sailing.

Your Stress and How to Manage It

What we perceive as stressful varies from person to person, as well as within the same person over time. Once you understand your own personal stress reactions and causes, you can learn to manage them. To be successful, stress management, like exercise, needs to be done regularly until it becomes a habit.

Research by behavioral scientists at Stanford and elsewhere has suggested that problem-solving strategies are effective in helping people manage stress in their lives. The problem-solving approach has five basic steps:

1. *Identify your major signs of stress.* Take a moment to think about this and use the chart entitled "Do You Have Any of These Signs of Stress?" to help you.

2. *Define your problem situations.* Sometimes simply stepping back and observing what we do can help identify problems that have gone unnoticed. Use the "Daily Stress and Tension Log" to help you with this.

3. *Develop possible solutions.* Some situations seem as if they are impossible to change. Take a little time to go through

Do You Have Any of These Signs of Stress?

Physical

Increased heart rate
Changes in breathing
Muscle tension
Tension headaches
Stomach/GI problems
Cold hands and/or feet
Sweaty palms
Hives, skin eruptions
Increased perspiration
Fatigue
Shakiness
Other: _____

Mental-Emotional

Difficulty concentrating
Distractibility
Narrowing of focus
Anxiety, nervousness
Moodiness, depression
Self-deprecatory thoughts
Irritability, anger
Other: _____

Behavioral

Increased arguing
Increased crying
Social withdrawal
Sleep changes
Changes in appetite
Poor performance
Changes in health habits
Voice changes
Other: _____

the stressful situations you note on your log and think about how you can avoid, alter, or adapt to the situation.

4. *Pick a strategy and put it into action.* If you think you might have trouble sticking to your new behavior, use a contract for change like the one shown here to help you.

5. *Evaluate how you are doing.* Answer these questions honestly: Is my stress-reduction strategy working? If so, how? If not, why not? Do I need a different strategy?

How Exercise Can Help Reduce Stress

Taking a walk is one of the items in the contract for change shown on page 48. And for a very good reason: A growing body of evidence indicates that physical activity may be able to counter the negative emotional effects of stress and be a significant aid in stress management.

William P. Morgan, a renowned sports psychologist, has documented that world-class athletes score below the general population on traits associated with anxiety, depression, anger, fatigue, and confusion, and above the general population on vigor. Similar results have been observed in nonathletic individuals who have been involved in a regular exercise program.

There is other evidence that exercise can reduce depression. In a Stanford study on men who recovered from heart attacks, 13 percent were moderately to severely depressed after their heart attack. Those who were placed on a regimen involving medically supervised exercise training showed a significant reduction on one measure of depression, compared to a control group. Of course, it is hard to generalize from this type of study; the fact that the men found themselves fit

Daily Stress and Tension Log

Use this log to keep track of your stressful situations on a daily basis. In the "Stress Rating" column, use a rating scale from 1 to 7, with 1 = very relaxed and 7 = very stressed.

Stress or Tensions Felt	Date and Time	Stress Rating	Where? Doing What? With Whom?	Thoughts/ Feelings	Response to Stress

enough to exercise at all could have been responsible for much of their improvement.

However, other studies support the hypothesis that physical activity and exercise probably help alleviate some of the symptoms associated with mild to moderate depression. There is also evidence that exercise is valuable in substance-abuse programs, reducing symptoms of anxiety and improving self-image.

In fact, the question of whether or not exercise has an antidepressive, calming effect may depend on the setting and the circumstances. At the very least, physical activity can provide

Contract for Change

Responsibilities:

For the next two weeks, as an aid to managing my stress levels, I will do the following:

1. Let my coworkers know the specific times during the day when I will be unavailable for questions or other interruptions. As an additional prompt, I will place a "Do Not Disturb" sign on my door during those times.

2. Defer any questions or problems during those designated periods to my coworker, *(his or her name here)*, as we have previously agreed. I will evaluate this work plan by recording the number of interruptions during those times.

3. Go for a walk after work at least three times during each week, as a way of helping me to unwind. I will evaluate my walking goal by noting the number of times I walked on my home calendar.

I will reevaluate these goals in two weeks.

Signed: _____

Work helper: _____

Home helper: _____

Date: _____

valuable "time out," during which the normal stresses of the day will cease. It can also enhance this time out by enabling people to enjoy positive, soothing experiences such as music, nature, the weather, or good conversation—which may be as beneficial as the exercise itself.

Exercise can also have the benefit of making people feel that they are taking charge of their health. This alone can be useful in stress reduction, and for psychological well-being in general. Moreover, there is evidence that aerobic training may be of value in reducing the physiological effects of stress.

In a study conducted through the Veterans Administration Medical Center at Jackson, Mississippi, in collaboration with the University of Mississippi, men with somewhat elevated blood pressure were observed as they underwent the stress of an exciting video game. Those men who had undergone aerobic exercise training showed a significantly smaller rise in blood pressure than that experienced by the men who had no such training. In other words, it appears that, for at least some people, exercise may lessen the damage that could otherwise be caused by the sudden rises in blood pressure resulting from unavoidable stress.

Physical activity is an excellent way to help you cope with the stress of your life. It provides an opportunity to leave daily stresses behind and focus your energies and thoughts on something positive. The physical and psychological benefits of exercise are great:

- a decrease in tension and anxiety
- an increase in feelings of well-being
- an increased capacity to do work

How to Take the Fun Out of Exercise

Under certain circumstances, an exercise session may be far from serene, and may even increase your level of anxiety. How can this possibly happen? Two words: scheduling and competition.

Scheduling. In an ideal world, you would find an otherwise free stretch of time in which to take your exercise, or would cancel a less important activity in order to make room for it. For many people, it doesn't work like that. Instead of replacing something on their schedule, they add exercise to it. If the schedule is already full, the addition of exercise to it may well produce considerable anxiety. "I'll never get this work done in time to get out of here!" "What if we get to the racquetball place and don't get a court?"

Competition. If you add to these tensions by engaging in competitive exercise like tennis or racquetball, and especially if winning is very important to you, your exercise session may be about as soothing as a plane wreck.

For some people, even less competitive forms of activity such as bicycling or running can produce great tension under certain circumstances. A crowded running track or a bicycle lane on a bus route can bring out depressingly hostile sides to the nature of otherwise reasonable people.

If you've been sedentary for a while, and don't believe any of this, I have one suggestion for you: Try it yourself. Take a walk with a friend, do some gardening, get out and about. I'll bet you're feeling calmer already!

Sittercise™: Exercises You Can Do Anywhere

Seated exercises can easily be done anywhere to help maintain comfort and improve overall fitness. They are especially helpful for use in relieving tight muscles at work or when traveling, and to help reduce specific back and neck pain, stiffness, and other discomfort caused by sitting. You can do seated exercises at your desk, in your car, on an airplane—anywhere you sit!

Do selected seated exercises throughout the day to ease the strain and discomfort of sitting for extended periods of time. Just two minutes of stretching during every hour of your work day adds up to over fifteen valuable minutes of tension-relieving stretches or muscle strengthening. Remember to stretch each muscle and joint slowly through its complete range of motion.

Ready? Here are some points to remember:

- To begin, sit comfortably in your chair with both feet resting on the floor and your back away from the backrest. Be sure the chair is secure.

- Keep your abdominal muscles contracted to help provide support for your lower back. Be careful not to slouch or arch your back.

- Breathe regularly and deeply. One of the most common mistakes is to hold your breath for the duration of any exercise. This makes the movement more difficult without increasing its effectiveness. You should do the movement and breathe at the same time—lightly inhale through your nose and exhale through your mouth several times as you hold the exercise.

- Especially if you work at a computer, remember that *preventive* action is important in helping reduce your risks of a repetitive-strain injury. Taking regular, planned stretch breaks at your desk helps reduce the risk factors involved in sustained posture and excessive duration.

- Do each movement slowly and deliberately, holding for fifteen to thirty seconds to fully stretch and relax.

NECK STRETCH *Relieves neck and upper-back tension.* Slowly lower your right ear to your right shoulder. Hold fifteen to thirty seconds, then slowly roll your head around to the left shoulder, keeping your chin close to your chest as you rotate. Repeat on left side. *Do not* make a complete circle or drop your head back on spine.

HAMSTRING STRETCH *Stretches hamstrings (back of upper thigh).* Sit forward on chair with your left leg bent and right leg extended forward. Keeping your seat firmly on the chair and bending from the hips, gently lean forward until you feel the stretch in the back of your leg. Straighten your leg as far as comfortable. Hold at least ten seconds. Repeat with left leg.

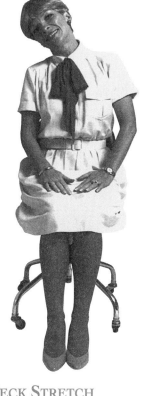

NECK STRETCH
Slowly lower your right ear to your right shoulder. Hold. Then slowly roll head to left shoulder, keeping chin close to chest. *Do not* make a complete circle or drop head back on spine.

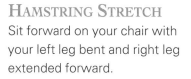

HAMSTRING STRETCH
Sit forward on your chair with your left leg bent and right leg extended forward.

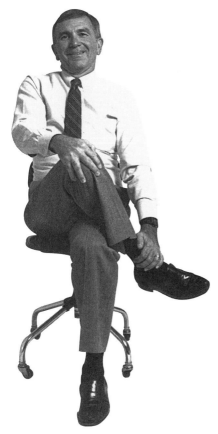

BOTTOM STRETCH   *Stretches buttock muscles; especially beneficial for airplane travel.* Cross your right leg over the left. Place your left hand on your shin, right hand on your knee. Gently pull the leg across and up toward your left shoulder. Then sit up as straight as possible, until you feel the stretch across your right buttock and leg.

OVERHEAD STRETCH AND HOLD

Stretches shoulder, upper back, and chest. Raise both arms over your head and reach high for the ceiling, trying to lift your upper body up and away from the rib cage. Avoid arching your lower back as arms lift. Hold at least ten seconds. Clasp hands overhead. Bring your elbows as close to your ears as possible; then pull arms back behind ears. Hold at least ten seconds.

BOTTOM STRETCH
Cross your right leg over the left, placing left hand on shin, right hand on knee. Gently pull leg up and across, and sit "up."

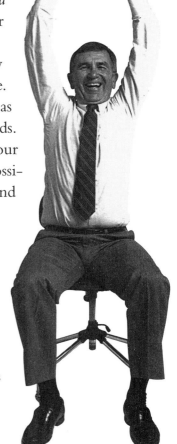

OVERHEAD STRETCH AND HOLD
Clasp hands overhead. Bring your elbows as close to your ears as possible; then pull arms back behind ears. Hold at least ten seconds.

Reducing Stress with the Mind-Body Approach

In addition to physical activity, an equally large and growing body of research indicates that various forms of passive relaxation—deep breathing, yoga, progressive relaxation, hypnosis, auto-hypnosis, autogenic training, and various forms of meditation—offer extensive physical and mental benefits. But stress often seems unrelenting and complex, while such relaxation strategies appear to be just too simple to really be effective.

How is it possible to even begin to resolve such a formidable issue? Or, as one patient asked, "So what do I do on Monday?" A great deal is possible. For better or for worse, the initial steps are quite simple: Establish a way to quiet your body and mind and establish an inner point of stillness from which you can examine and change negative, destructive thoughts and behaviors. Unfortunately, the means to this end are often expressed in either of two extremes: in esoteric meditation practice or in overly simplistic forms of the power of positive thinking. Neither extreme is viable, and both tend to turn off more people than they motivate.

TEN PRACTICAL STEPS TO QUIET THE BODY AND MIND

Between these two extremes, however, is a highly effective approach based on three steps: quieting the body, quieting the mind, and using this state of inner balance to visualize alternatives.

It's not necessary to understand the underlying biology to effectively follow these steps, but a few insights may be helpful. During the physical quieting step, the focus is on the two sensations of "heaviness" and "warmth." Heaviness is the subjective sensation of muscles relaxing, while warmth is the subjective sensation of increased blood flow to the periphery of the body, into the hands and feet, as an indication of overall relaxation. By focusing on these two sensations, you are essentially asking or communicating with both the voluntary muscle system of the body as well as the supposedly involuntary, or smooth muscles of the circulatory system. In both cases, the purpose is to quiet the body and become fully free of the usual physical tensions and distractions that are an inevitable part of everyday life.

These are ten practical steps to quiet the body and mind:

1. Choose a comfortable, armless, straight-backed chair such as a kitchen table chair. Sit comfortably on the chair toward the front edge, so that your back is not resting against the back of the chair. This is a posture of balance that will keep you from becoming drowsy or falling asleep as you do this for longer periods of time. Just let your arms and hands hang straight down by your sides.

2. Gently close your eyes and focus your full attention on the act of sitting in a relaxed and balanced posture. While in this position, slide the left foot forward until you feel your weight shift to your heel. Then slide the foot back in toward your body until you begin to feel your weight pressing on the ball of your foot. Moving your foot in this manner, find the position in which your foot is flat on the floor with your weight evenly distributed on both the heel and the ball of your foot. In this position, your leg should be extended in front of you approximately at a 120-degree angle. Then do the same thing with your right foot. There should be no ten-

Myth: Exercise is stressful for the body.

Fact: Exercise dissolves stress, helps you relax, and gives you energy to better handle stressful situations.

> "Ask anyone who exercises if it helps them cope with stress and they'll say, 'Yes, of course.' Like them, exercise is one of my primary forms of stress relief." —Terrie Rizzo

sion in the legs, and the knees should be approximately one foot apart. Hold your knees in your hands and wriggle them so that your legs move without resistance.

3. Now that your legs are in a stable position and you are balanced between the soles of your feet and the base of your spine, you can balance the upper part of your body as well. Moving the upper part of your body as though it was one unit, just lean forward until you feel your lower back muscles pulling. Then allow yourself to lean back in the chair until you feel your abdominal muscles pulling. Next, as you did with your feet, rock back and forth until you find the position where neither set of muscles is strained and the spinal column feels as if it is poised perfectly on the pelvis. This means the torso is in a state of balance.

4. Next, turn your attention to your head and drop your head forward onto your chest until the muscles at the back of your neck pull. Rock your head back and forth until it feels like a ball balanced on the end of your spinal column, which is in turn balanced on your pelvis.

5. Muscles generally need to be tensed in order to rebound and relax maximally. Because back and neck muscles carry a great deal of tension, it is best to tense and relax these muscle groups. To do this, just imagine that there is a string from the top of your head to the ceiling and that this string is pulling you into an upright posture with both arms still hanging down to the sides. Then imagine that the string is cut and your head just flops forward like a rag doll. It is very important that you not collapse over your throat, which would make breathing difficult.

Myth: You only reap the benefits of exercise if you stick to your program come hell or high water.

Fact: The key to an effective program is to listen to your body and know what level and type of exercise is right for you each day.

6. While you are sitting in this relaxed position, just raise your left hand and let it drop on your thigh as if it were a dead weight. Do the same with your right hand and let them both relax where they fall.

7. Then just let your attention flow like water down into your left arm and hand. Silently say to yourself, "My left arm is heavy and warm." There is no magic in those worlds, they are simply meant to remind you to feel these two sensations. Repeat this phrase three times. As during any relaxation meditation practice, your mind may tend to stray as you attempt to focus on the exercise, but there is no need to be disturbed by this. Merely direct your attention back to the task at hand in a gentle manner without getting upset at your vagrant imagination or trying too hard to hold your focus.

8. Then let your attention flow up to your head and face and silently repeat, "My face feels cool." This is to direct blood flow away from the head and face and out to the extremities, a signal to the body and mind to become increasingly relaxed. Again repeat this phrase three times. You might imagine a cool breeze blowing over your face from the ocean or from the mountains.

9. Finally, let your attention flow down into your right arm and hand and silently repeat, "My right arm is heavy and warm" three times. At this point, you are in a state of being physically relaxed and mentally alert. In order to make it increasingly easy to achieve this state of quiet, it is helpful to take a mental picture of your position, the feelings of heaviness and warmth, and overall posture so that it becomes clear and familiar. It is like creating a map of how to get to a famil-

iar destination, and the more you visit this place the easier it becomes to find.

10. Ending is as important as beginning. Time for this practice can range anywhere from two to fifteen minutes and will usually lengthen as you practice. Take a deep breath and as you do, raise your hands up toward your chest. As you exhale, stretch your legs, stand up, or do whatever you want in order to feel how good it is to move after sitting still for so long.

We all differ in our ability to succeed at relaxation, and the help of a trained therapist is always useful in monitoring progress and determining at what point to move on to your next step. However, the sensations of heaviness will be very real to you when you are doing the exercises correctly. You will not feel that they are just imaginary. This will tell you that you are mastering the practice. It all sounds deceptively simple, but it can bring a pronounced positive effect to your entire body and mind.

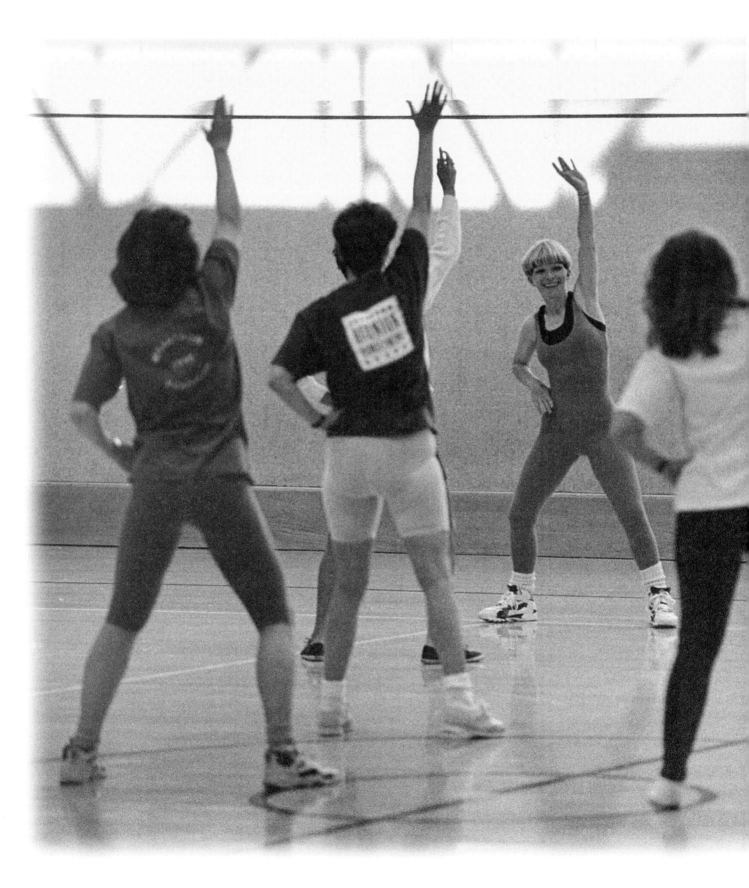

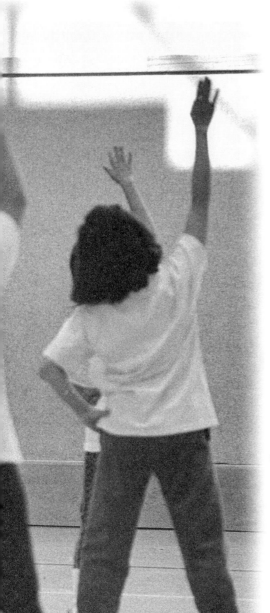

Part Two

Get Started Now!

"Why wait to begin leading an active life? Exercise is a great way to have fun and use your body throughout the day. Many daily activities count as exercise— walking your dog, gardening, taking the stairs instead of the elevator. When you start thinking this way, you'll be off to a fresh start."

—Terrie Rizzo

No
Excuses!

June A. Flora, PH.D.

People can come up with an array of excuses for not exercising that are quite breathtaking in their ingenuity and diversity. What's yours?

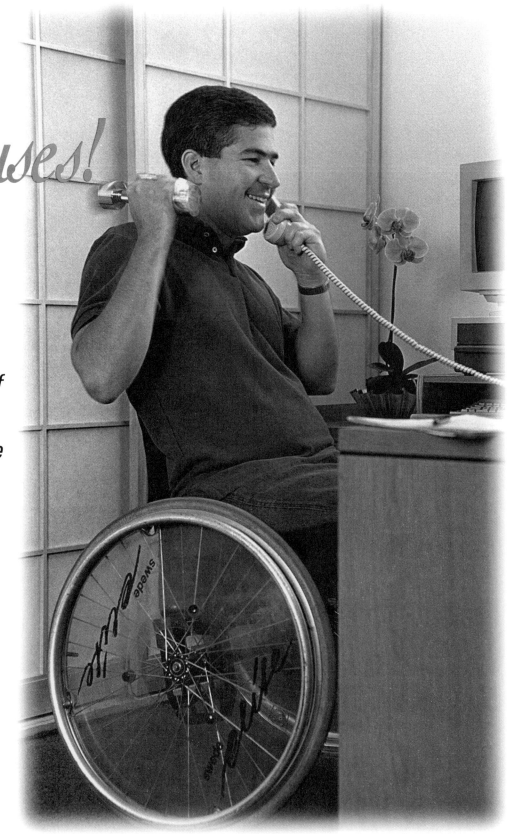

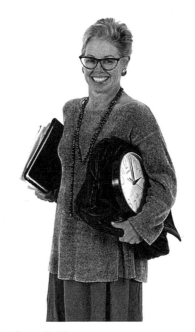

EOPLE WHO HAVE BEEN EXERCISING regularly for a few months tend to become hooked: They wouldn't quit if you paid them to. But getting started, and staying with exercise for the first critical months, may not be easy. Indeed, people can come up with an array of excuses that are quite breathtaking in their ingenuity and diversity. Unfortunately, these excuses may develop into permanent barriers unless they are confronted and systematically dismantled.

If you have not yet started exercising, or have quit, you will probably find some of your own excuses here. First, take this simple diagnostic test. Then read the appropriate sections that will help you find ways to overcome your own personal barriers.

June A. Flora, PH.D., is Associate Director of the Stanford Center for Research in Disease Prevention. For exercise, she enjoys jogging and aerobics.

Category T: Time Management

If you have trouble finding time for exercise, you are not alone. But even if the prospect of extracting thirty minutes out of your day seems daunting (forty if you include the shower), it is probably not impossible. To overcome the notion that there are not enough hours in the day, consider the following four strategies:

1. *Get up earlier.* If possible, add time to your day by exercising early in the morning, when the world is beautiful. You may find that waking forty minutes or an hour earlier three days a week proves surprisingly easy to manage. Although your hours in bed may be reduced, the quality of your sleep may more than make up for it—regular exercise helps many to fall asleep more easily and sleep more soundly.

Self-Test: What's Your Excuse?

Some of these statements apply to people who have not yet started to exercise, and some apply to people who started but quit. Check off all the statements that apply to you.

1. I am afraid that exercise will make me look silly. **(C)**

2. I exercised for a while, then stopped when I went on vacation. **(A)**

3. I exercised, but it never felt easy or pleasant. **(P)**

4. I will exercise sometime—when I can get my outfit color-coordinated. **(K)**

5. I quit because I didn't seem to be improving. **(R)**

6. People often laughed at me when I expressed enthusiasm for exercise. **(S)**

7. Exercise hurt: My muscles were always sore. **(P)**

8. I only exercised because my spouse/ doctor wanted me to. **(W)**

9. I don't have time. **(T)**

10. I think exercise will increase my appetite, and I will put on weight. **(M)**

11. I get very tired and/or short of breath when I exercise. **(P)**

12. I felt I would never be as thin (or agile) as the others in the class/group. **(R)**

13. I simply disliked every type of exercise I have tried. **(W)**

14. I am afraid I might have a heart attack. **(M)**

15. I will exercise when I move closer to my work/when the kids grow up/ when I get a different job. **(T)**

16. I don't like to exercise alone. **(S)**

17. I can't decide which exercise to try. **(K)**

18. I used to exercise but stopped when I got sick **(A)**

19. (For women): I am afraid of developing large muscles. **(M)**

20. I didn't like the people in the class/ group. **(S)**

21. I think exercise is a fad, and people will laugh at me for being fashionable. **(C)**

22. I would exercise if the day were an hour longer. **(T)**

23. I quit because I never achieved my goals. **(R)**

24. I tried exercising and was sore for a week. **(P)**

25. I was just getting started when some relatives came to stay or the weather turned bad or something. **(A)**

Scoring: Add up the letters, and write the totals here:

T:_____ W:_____ R:_____ S:_____ P:_____ K:_____ M:_____ A:_____ C:_____

If you scored points in any category, read the appropriate section.

2. *Double up your activities.* Exercise and do something else at the same time. For example:

- Read the paper, dictate memos, or watch the television news while you are on your exercise bicycle.

- Listen to tapes of meetings while you walk or jog.

- Arrange to conduct important conversations with family or colleagues while you walk.

3. *Get some help.* If you can afford it, hire someone to do something you would otherwise be spending time on (yard work, housecleaning, child watching, car cleaning) and exercise during that time. It makes the exercise sessions difficult to forget or skip.

4. *Simply make time for exercise.* "Impossible!" you exclaim? Then complete this exercise. In an average week, could you find time to do three of the following? Check the ones you would not find excuses to avoid:

- Stand in the street for half an hour to watch your baseball team parade by after it has won the World Series.

- Drive to school to talk to your child's teacher.

- Pick up your child at the airport.

- Go to a godchild's wedding.

- Watch your neighbor's slides of his European vacation.

- Attend a protest meeting about a new high-rise to be built in your neighborhood.

- Shop for your spouse's anniversary present.

Finished? Since the chance of all those demands on your time coming up this week is remote, you have probably just

Eight Ways to Avoid Excuses

1. Be creative about finding time to exercise.

2. Think ahead about possible interruptions to your exercise program and plan ways to minimize or avoid them.

3. Find people you like to exercise with.

4. Set realistic exercise goals.

5. Find an exercise that genuinely entertains you.

6. Don't start an exercise program until you're ready to make a commitment to keep it up.

7. Understand your physical limitations and exercise appropriately.

8. Don't exercise with people who make you feel self-conscious.

liberated three periods of time for exercise. However, don't rely on the chance of finding an empty stretch of time and deciding at the last minute to fill it with exercise. That seldom works. For most people, some planning is essential: Decide when you will exercise, and write it down—preferably where others can see it and remind you of it, gently, if you forget.

Category A: You Accidentally Quit

The A scale describes those who "accidentally" stopped exercising. Perhaps you stopped exercising when you went on vacation, when your mother-in-law came to visit, when you attended a conference, or when you got the flu. It happens all the time. Fortunately, you can get out of the habit of accidentally quitting with some simple techniques.

EXCUSE: I GOT SICK   If you get sick, realize the danger of sedentary relapse (which could be more hazardous to your health than your current ailment) and use any part of your brain that can still function to try and avoid it. For example, if you exercise with a friend, tell him or her what day you can reasonably expect to be recovered and go back to your routine. Don't rush it: Expect to spend a week or so on your own getting back into shape by walking before you resume vigorous exercise. But making that commitment ahead of time will prevent a slide into inactivity.

EXCUSE: I WAS OUT OF TOWN ON BUSINESS   If you are to go on a business trip, find out ahead of time what the exercise facilities are. In addition, business associates or conference organizers are now used to such requests, and can give you information on jogging trails, swimming pools, or access to health club facilities. Many hotels have their own gyms for guests.

EXCUSE: I WENT ON VACATION   Before you go on vacation, think ahead about its potential for keeping your body in reasonable shape—not necessarily through regular exercise sessions, but as an incidental part of the trip. Try to include at least one activity every day or so that will keep your whole body moving around briskly for twenty minutes or more without stopping. If this activity doesn't happen to be supplied by a volleyball game, or a game of tennis, or body-surfing, or skiing, or a mountain hike, or sightseeing in a foreign city with no parking places or public transportation, then make a point of adding a fast walk at least once every other day. It won't spoil your vacation, and it will keep your muscles and cardiovascular system primed for your return.

EXCUSE: I HAD TO ENTERTAIN MY RELATIVES   If social commitments at home, such as visits from relatives, tend to push exercise habits to the back burner (from which they never recover), then plan your strategy well before the visit. Guests should understand that exercise now constitutes an immovable part of your household's routine. If some commitment makes it impossible for you to take part in your normal exercise routine for a week or so, at least plan mini-sessions, or walks, to tide you over.

Category M: Myths

People with category M excuses wrongly believe in the exercise myths you'll find throughout this book. Exercise need not provoke heart attacks, increase weight, make women look masculine, or any of the many other things people wrongly believe. The best way around this obstacle is solid information: See the chapters Why Exercise Works and Change Your Life with Exercise.

Myth: Regular exercise means devoting many hours every week to working out.

Fact: With a little planning, you can weave extra activity right into your daily routine.

Category S: Social Support

If you scored in category S, here's a simple solution to your exercise problems: Find the right kind of people to do it with. Some exercisers relish solitude (and in some cases, as when there is only one exercise bicycle at home, they have little choice). However, if your sport and your schedule can be adapted to include others, your chances of persisting will be greatly enhanced. Exercising with others has a number of additional advantages:

- It will make time go faster.
- It will help you go about your exercise in a sensible way—without excesses.
- It will instill a mildly competitive spirit.
- It will provide a supportive group of people who will immediately understand your problems, share your aches, and fully appreciate your accomplishments.

It's up to you if you'd rather join a formal group or exercise with one or more friends and colleagues on an informal basis. If your temperament is suited to leadership, you could ensure your own consistency in exercise by setting up a group yourself! While you will help others, you will be the main beneficiary, finding it impossible to let your own exercise routine lapse, except at the risk of letting others down.

Category R: Realistic Expectations

If you scored high on the R scale, you could use a dose of realism. You are expecting either too much or too little of yourself, and it is interfering with the reality of what you can actually do. Most people can improve steadily in both strength and stamina if they stick to their exercise program consistently. Few people, however, can run marathons in their second week—and some should never think of running marathons at all.

As you will see from other chapters in this book, even the best natural athletes should start their program gradually; the older you are, and the longer you have been sedentary, the longer it will take to get back in shape. And you will never be as fast/graceful/strong as the athlete twenty or thirty years younger.

By all means, if you are a goal-setting person, set goals. For example, decide that one year from now you will enter a 10K race and finish it. But if you are new to exercise, don't set your sights on the race next week or even next month. In the early stages, at least, set goals in terms of time rather than speed or distance. Plan to run/walk/swim an extra ten minutes, at the appropriate heart rate: You can't fail.

Category W: Something's Seriously Wrong

Category W responses could signal the need for serious rethinking. Perhaps you tried exercise only because you were ordered to do so; perhaps you have no serious intention of ever trying to enjoy it. Perhaps you have found it very boring.

You are not yet giving up on the whole idea of exercise (if you were, you would not be reading this book), but you are thinking about it. And it's certainly a good idea to try to bypass your problems with exercise.

EXCUSE: I'LL NEVER RUN A MARATHON Approach the subject from a new angle. Don't think in terms of exercise, but of getting your heart rate up to a respectable beat three times a week for twenty minutes, no matter how you do it.

EXCUSE: EXERCISE IS BORING Consider forms of "play" that would genuinely entertain you, and also raise your heart rate—inline skating, ice-skating, skiing, surfing, square dancing, Scottish country dancing, soccer, basketball. Check out everything you can do safely while watching television or listening to a book on tape or music on headphones: walking, running, stationary cycling, walking up and down your stairs.

EXCUSE: I HATE SPORTS Think of all the things you could do, and perhaps are doing anyway, that are exercise in disguise: housework or yard work, walking to lunch, cleaning the car. Upgrade those jobs to make them brisk enough to raise your heart rate to the appropriate range (see the chapter Creating Your Own Exercise Program) and keep them going

> "It's easy to make excuses for not exercising. The trick is to find ways to be more active!"
> —Terrie Rizzo

for the appropriate length of time. If you can fit in two of those a week, and add one long weekend walk, you can count yourself as an exerciser.

Category K: Who Are You Trying to Kid?

If you had K responses, you are not yet ready to risk trying to become a serious exerciser. Your commitment, at most, is wobbly. It may be best to postpone any idea of a regular exercise program right now. Without a serious commitment, you might tend to quit after a few sessions and let that failure inhibit you from trying on later occasions.

Better wait until you feel that you have the time, the social support, the right color socks…and a serious intention of starting an exercise program that you will maintain. Then start with the suggestions in category W.

Category P: Physical Problems

If you checked one or more P answers, you quit exercising because of physical difficulties. There is probably no need to give up all idea of exercise (almost everyone with feet—and indeed without them—can do something), but it would be wise to learn what's at the root of your problems.

- If you had any pains in the chest, extreme shortness of breath, or tiredness long after stopping the exercise, tell your doctor.

- If exercise made your limbs or joints ache, read the chapter Don't Hurt Yourself! You probably tried to do too much too soon, with insufficient stretching and perhaps the wrong shoes.

Few people can simply take their bodies out of storage after twenty or thirty years of idleness, dust them off, wind them up, and expect that all the parts will still mesh like a well-tuned machine. Next time, treat your body more gently by starting slowly. Expect some minor muscle aches, and expect also to feel physically tired at the end of your exercise session. But don't exercise so vigorously that these symptoms will persist, or interfere seriously with the smooth running of your life.

Category C: You Feel Conspicuous

If you checked one or more C answers, you feel self-conscious. You feel people are laughing at you for following the exercise fad, or for looking unathletic.

There may, in fact, be no reason for your self-consciousness, but it can be an inhibiting feeling whether justified or not, and it is worth taking seriously. Here are some solutions:

- Exercise at home (for example, on an exercise bicycle) until you are too athletic-looking to be laughed at.
- Join a health club or class with people who are in the same shape you are.
- Walk. To avoid all charges of affectation or faddishness, get a dog to walk with you.

Eventually, exercise will become more important to you than self-consciousness. You honestly won't care what people think, and they will admire and envy you for it.

Your Exercise Tool Kit

A few years ago, we conducted an interesting project about exercise. One of our more ambitious aims was to get the populations of Salinas and Monterey, California, on their feet and exercising. Through booklets, newspaper articles, TV spots and programs, worksite contests, neighborhood organizations, fun runs, and school-based programs, we urged people in these communities to get out there and do something aerobic.

Many of them did, and they gave us glowing testimonials about the changes exercise had made in their lives. But many failed to respond to our urging. Or they responded for a week or so, then went back to watching television. Even though we had convinced them of the benefits of exercise, we had evidently not given them sufficient tools to overcome the exercise barriers in their path.

Our greatest success was with a program that did give people the tools they needed to overcome those barriers. This was a self-help "Walking Kit" that got them started slowly, and held their hands every step of the way. We suggest that you follow some of the main principals of that program:

1. Make a commitment (to yourself or to others) that you will exercise regularly for a period of at least several weeks.

2. Start slowly: Stay well within your capacity.

3. Do all you can to make the experience sociable, enjoyable, and relaxing.

4. Be aware of situations that might lead to a relapse, and take steps to avoid them.

After a few months, if all goes well, you should be hooked. Then you'll be able to look back with astonishment at the sort of wild excuses you once created to avoid this deeply pleasurable activity.

Don't *Hurt* Yourself!

Donald M. Bunce, M.D.
Standley L. Scott, P.T., A.T.C.
Tim N. Bowman, M.S., P.T., A.T.C.

The leading cause of athletic injuries can be summed up simply: Too much, too soon.

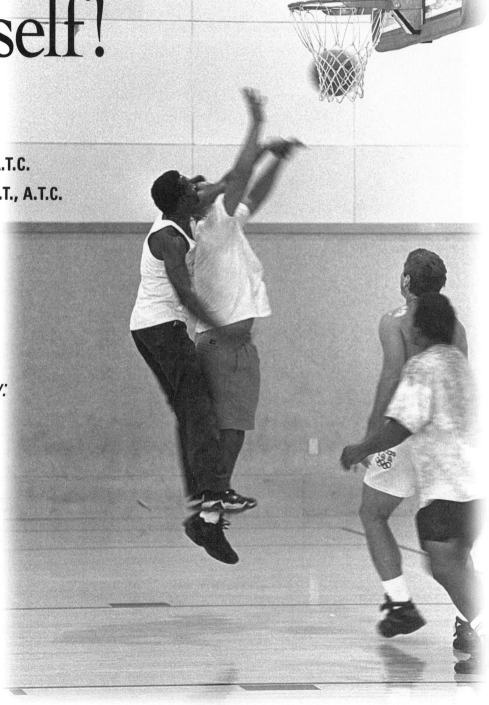

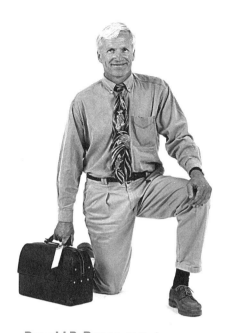

Donald R. Bunce, M.D., is Clinical Associate Professor in the Department of Orthopedics, and an orthopedic surgeon with the Palo Alto Medical Clinic. He is team physician for Stanford University and the San Francisco Giants. He regularly participates in exercise he considers fun, such as tennis and paddleball.

A T THE STANFORD ATHLETIC DEPARTMENT'S Office of Athletic Training and Sports Medicine, we see 400 to 500 athletes each day, most with some degree of injury ranging from bruises, strains, and sprains to fractures, dislocations, and nerve injuries. We treat them and explain to the athletes how to avoid aggravating them further.

More than likely, we'll see them again—it's pretty hard for a young athlete in a full-contact sport to stay off the injured list. But for most exercisers, injuries are not inevitable. In fact, with some simple precautions, there's no reason to get injured at all.

Know Your Body

If you wanted to erect a house on a vacant piece of property, you'd consult with experts: a geologist, to make sure the land was stable, and an architect, to design the best structure for the site.

Improving your body is no different. Consulting with someone who understands your chosen activity and who can anticipate the long-term effects of the stresses it brings is crucial. Determining these effects is the best way to prevent athletic injuries.

If you have heart disease, arthritis, diabetes, lower-back pain, and other conditions that can prevent you from participating in some activities, your doctor can best determine your medical fitness. If you have had previous bone, muscle, or joint injuries, or a postural defect, an orthopedist's advice would be valuable as well.

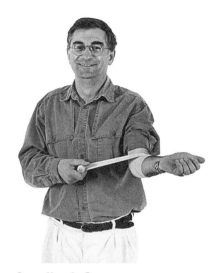

Standley L. Scott, P.T., A.T.C, is the athletic trainer for all Stanford varsity sports, and was on the medical staff of the 1984 Olympic Games. He is also a faculty adviser for the Stanford Human Biology Program. He regularly runs, bikes, and does stair-climbing and cross-country skiing machines.

If you are generally healthy, however, you can determine your physical fitness by performing the self-tests provided in this book or by consulting a physical therapist, certified athletic trainer, exercise physiologist, or physical educator. Ideally, these professionals can evaluate your existing condition and recommend programs that will allow you to proceed with your preferred activity.

Physical defects that don't affect the routines of daily living can be magnified greatly once you intensify your level of activity. Running, for instance, magnifies the stress on your feet five to eight times that of walking. For ballistic sports—anything that involves high-velocity contact with a ball using a bat, a racket, or your foot—it's important to determine whether your body parts can withstand the intensity of impact.

Commonly existing conditions such as having one leg longer than the other, high or low arches, knock-knees, or bowleggedness should all be identified. Special attention should be paid to the patello-femoral joint around the kneecap, the site of many athletic injuries.

If you have these or other physical deviations, it may be wise to seek advice on athletic activities that may be less stressful for you than the exercise you were planning. Just because everyone else is running doesn't mean that you have to run as well; bicycling, swimming, and walking can be just as beneficial and enjoyable.

Overuse Syndrome: Too Much, Too Soon

As the body adapts itself to the stresses of exercise, overuse can occur in almost any body tissue: muscles, joints, or bones. You probably know someone who has suffered an acute overload injury such as tennis elbow, shinsplints, heel spurs, fractures, dislocations, ligament sprains, or muscle pulls. These injuries occur when you put more stress on a body part than it can handle, and it breaks, tears, or twists. These injuries are painful, but they generally go away with treatment. When you ignore injuries, however, they can become chronic and far more difficult to treat.

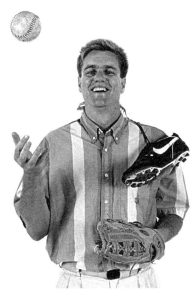

Tim N. Bowman, M.S., P.T., A.T.C., has been a physical therapist and athletic trainer for over fifteen years, and is Director of the Physical Therapy Department at Stanford University's Student Health Center. He enjoys hiking, inline skating, and basketball.

WHO IS AT RISK?   Who is at risk of developing overload injury? Mostly older athletes, people who have been injured before, and those in poor condition.

The older exerciser. As the aging process occurs, most of the connective tissue of our bodies—tendons, ligaments, fascia—become weaker and somewhat less elastic, resulting in more frequent overload injuries. Rarely do very young athletes pull muscles, or develop chronic tendinitis, fasciitis, or bursitis.

Women beyond the age of menopause are at high risk of developing osteoporosis—bones that are more susceptible to stress fractures even with moderate activity. Exercise in moderation, hormone replacement, and sometimes vitamin D, calcium supplements, and fluoride may minimize this risk. Postmenopausal women with osteoporosis may want to seek the advice of an internist or endocrinologist before exercising. Recently, as we'll see later in this chapter, research has found that weight-bearing exercise—including swimming—can help build denser bones no matter how old you are.

Previous injuries. People who have previously been in-

> "If you resist the temptation to overdo it, you'll prevent most injuries. But if something hurts, deal with it immediately. Use common sense and never ignore pain."
> —Terrie Rizzo

jured are also at risk. Often the rest required to heal a previous injury will result in some degree of muscle atrophy and bone weakness; as a result, those structures may become overloaded when training resumes.

Those in poor condition, therefore, are particularly vulnerable to injury. If you return to a sport such as skiing and your thigh strength is poor, you are susceptible to muscle fatigue, which can result in serious injury to the cartilage and ligaments of the knee and bones of the legs.

Connective-tissue problems. People who are considered "connective-tissue sensitive" are also at risk. These are people who may have early rheumatology conditions. Recurring joint inflammations and tendinitis are common warning signals.

STRESS FRACTURES Stress fractures are small cracks in bone caused by repetitive stresses, weight-bearing in the lower extremities, and stress on bone from muscle attachments in the upper extremities. They are similar to "fatigue failure" of metal after it has been stressed thousands of times. The difference between bone and metal, or course, is that bone is a dynamic living tissue that has the ability to repair itself.

Stress fractures seldom lead to complete breaks because pain often stops the athlete from continuing at an injurious pace. Stress fractures are extremely common in the novice exerciser who rapidly increases the frequency, duration, intensity, or biomechanical aspects of a workout. You can develop stress or fatigue fractures in one weekend—again, too much, too soon, too hard—or over the course of a year, even if you're not in good shape.

Physical Stress Builds Bones

Under normal circumstances, bone is quite durable. Like muscle, it has the remarkable potential for remodeling—resuming its former size and shape. Bone responds to physical stress or the lack of it—new bone is deposited at sites of stress and reabsorbed from areas of little stress. The younger and more active the individual, the greater the potential for bone remodeling and growth. Genetics can also play a role. It has been known for some time that stress fractures are less common in athletes of African descent, whose bones may be thicker and stronger than those of whites.

A striking example of how bone weakens when it is not stressed is the effect of weightless environments on bones. It has been estimated that 25 percent of total body calcium can be lost in one year of space travel—about the time it takes to go from Earth to Mars. Other factors—physical stress, hormones (that is, estrogen), amount of dietary calcium, intestinal disease, vitamin D, ultraviolet light, and phosphorus—are all very important components of healthy bone metabolism. But physical stress is the only method known to increase bone mass regardless of age. Studies of animals and humans have reported denser, stronger, and usually thicker bones following exercise. More than any other method, exercise can strengthen and maintain healthy bones, countering the effects of injury and aging.

Myth: No pain, no gain.

Fact: Train! Don't strain.

An Ounce of Prevention . . .

The easiest way to prevent injury during exercise is to exercise properly. That means a good warm-up, a stretching routine, getting into your aerobic activity gradually, and cooling down afterward.

FIRST, WARM UP Until you warm up the body parts you intend to exercise, any activity is too much, too soon. A good warm-up readies your body for more intense activity, preparing the nerves, muscles, and joints. It increases the blood flow to the area in question, actually raising its temperature, expanding the tissue, making it more supple and easier to stretch. Blood flow also increases mechanical efficiency by delivering more nutrients and reducing friction. Increased oxygen flow enables the muscles to work harder.

Start your warm-up with brisk walking or slow jogging. Generally, when your body breaks into a sweat (usually about after five minutes of activity), you are ready for the next phase of warm-up: stretching.

NEXT, STRETCH Stretching should always come midway in the warm-up. If you stretch too soon, your muscles may not be supple enough. Stretching itself should be slow and relaxing, held at the point where you feel tightness within the muscle—never in the joint—for about thirty seconds. All stretches should be held for thirty seconds. If you feel the muscle relaxing, move an inch or so farther into the stretch. Your breathing should be relaxed and normal and the stretching done slowly. Don't bounce.

While your particular activity will dictate the best warm-up for you, almost all athletic pursuits involve muscle groups in the calf, the backs of the thighs (hamstrings), the back, and the abdomen. These areas almost always need to be warmed for optimal flexibility. For specific exercises, see the chapter on Stretching for Flexibility.

START SLOWLY The third stage of warm-up actually involves rehearsing your planned activity at a less intense level —do your first few tennis serves at 50 percent rather than "aces," work from a slow jog to a faster run, cycle at a slower pace and work up, and so on. If you throw yourself full force into your activity, even though you're warmed up and stretched, you run the risk of injury.

COOL DOWN BEFORE YOU STOP To prevent injury, a gradual cool-down at the end of your exercise is just as crucial as a pre-exercise warm-up. Gradually decrease the intensity of your activity to allow your system to return to a normal resting state slowly rather than abruptly. Spend five or ten minutes slowly walking or stretching to allow your body to remove lactic acid and other chemical waste products of exercise from your muscles, rather than allowing them to settle there. Abruptly ending exercise can also cause dizziness or fainting.

Use the Proper Equipment

If you think that proper equipment means only the right skis, the right tennis racquet, or the right bike, you have overlooked some very important items: your clothes, your shoes, and the exercise machines in your home or at your gym.

CLOTHES Dressing smart is easy. Don't allow yourself to be overheated because you're overclothed. Remember, your body

Old Favorites That Can Hurt You

One result of studying the long-term effects of exercise has been to expose some of the most time-honored exercises as harmful. If you have been doing any of the following old favorites, stop. If you've never done them, don't start!

1. The *duck walk*—waddling on your haunches—is actually detrimental to your knees. Any time you flex your knees, particularly with your full weight on them, you risk damaging them.

2. The *hurdler's stretch*—sitting with one leg straight in front and the other bent back at your side—puts undue pressure on the hip joint and the medial side of the knees.

3. *Straight leg raises*—lying flat on your back and lifting both legs—puts stress on the back and doesn't strengthen the muscles you might think it does.

4. *Straight-leg sit-ups*—lying flat on your back with legs extended and trying to do a sit-up—puts undue strain on the lower back and doesn't do much for the abdominals.

5. *Touching your toes while standing* doesn't stretch the hamstrings adequately and should be avoided because of possible stress on the back.

6. *Full neck circles* can grind down the vertebrae in your neck and spine.

7. *Grand pliés or deep squats* can damage your knees.

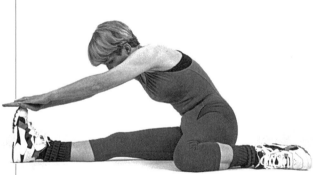

HURDLER'S STRETCH
This is a good way to damage your hips and knees.

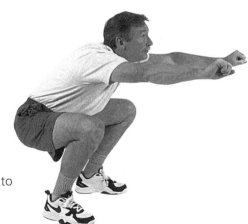

STRAIGHT-LEG SIT-UPS
This old standard is a great way to hurt your back!

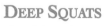

DEEP SQUATS
A quick and easy way to hurt your knees.

If the Shoe Fits

Whatever your activity, if the shoe doesn't fit, you may be in for trouble. Always buy athletic shoes according to your foot type, your activity (high or low impact), and your floor surface. Here are some more things to keep in mind:

- **Fit and comfort:** Make sure that the shoe is neither too narrow nor too wide, the arch is properly supported, the heel is snug, and the toes have plenty of room. Are there any pressure points?

- **Cushion:** Jump on the toes to test forefoot cushion; walk or jog slowly to judge rear-foot cushion. Note: Too much cushion can make a shoe less stable.

- **Stability:** Does your foot tend to roll to the inside or outside? Test forefoot stability by jumping on your toes, rear-foot stability by feeling if your heel rolls inward or outward. Evaluate lateral stability by jumping side to side to see if the shoe keeps your foot centered.

- **Flexibility:** Hold the heel and press the toe down on a flat surface. Does the shoe flex at the ball of the foot? When you're on the toes, is the heel firmly in place?

- **Outside traction:** Walk on a surface comparable to the floor or carpet you exercise on. Does the shoe glide and pivot well, or does it slip or snag?

Source: International Dance-Exercise Association, Inc. (IDEA).

needs some method of evaporation—even in cold weather—so always wear fabrics that breathe. Don't exercise in a heavy sweat suit or a rubber-coated suit that doesn't allow perspiration to escape into the air.

SHOES The most common equipment-related injury stems from a bad shoe fit. The mechanics of the foot and the entire leg are such that, improperly equipped, they can contribute to injuries—even those that are not foot-related. For instance, women are more susceptible to lower-extremity injuries than men because of the shape of the pelvis; the stresses on their hips, knees, and feet contribute to problems that incorrect shoes only aggravate.

Make sure your shoes fit properly and comfortably and give you adequate support. It also pays to make sure that you have the proper shoe for the activity you're doing. Don't run in court shoes, don't hike in running shoes, don't do aerobics in basketball shoes. Some cross-training shoes can do double duty. Buy your shoes (or at least try them on) at a store where the salespeople know what they're talking about.

If you have a pre-exercise physical examination, it should include your feet, particularly the arches. Lack of arch support can lead to significant injury. One common foot motion is called pronation—the flattening of the inside of the foot under weight. Pronation and hyperpronation can cause a chain reaction of problems all the way up the leg to the back, but good shoe fit can correct them.

MACHINES   If your athletic program is going to include home exercise equipment, mention this to your health-care professional. There's a wide variety of home equipment, most of which is very good. But again, any preexisting conditions you have need to be identified. If you have stiffness, tightness, or lack of motion from a previous injury, and couple it with the configuration of a piece of equipment, you may find yourself sitting or lying down in an unnatural position that creates additional problems for you. A previous injury to your patello-femoral joint (that is, underneath and around your kneecap), for instance, may prelude you from straightening your knee against resistance, as some equipment requires.

Use the concept of *progressive resistance exercise* with a machine. Increase the intensity of your exercise incrementally; when ten repetitions come easily, increase the number of reps, or the poundage. If you ease into a machine's use, and don't overdo, it's less likely that you will injure yourself. Most of the machines available are safe. For more on machines and how they work to strengthen muscles, see the chapter Why Exercise Works.

Identifying an Injury

If you do sustain an injury, you need to know how to identify it and keep it from getting worse.

PAIN Defining an injury is difficult because you're dealing with pain, which is very subjective. Some people can tune out pain, others will deny it. The important thing is to discern the difference between pain and discomfort. You have to be able to differentiate between the feeling of having worked hard and a consistently recurring pain that comes on every repetition of a motion; the latter is a good warning sign that something's awry.

Pain can also communicate that more rest is needed between intense workouts, that you should go more slowly, or that you haven't recovered from a previous injury. An interval of rest is just as important as the exercise itself. Your soreness must subside before you exercise again; it's crucial that you don't try to work through the pain.

The method we often use with young athletes is to have them describe the quality of pain and rate it on a scale of one to ten. Muscle soreness can manifest itself at rest, after you've exercised, and that's no cause for concern. But if you have an aching pain that keeps you awake or even wakes you from sleep, it should be investigated. If you find yourself taking an undue amount of pain medication, too, seek professional medical advice. Dizziness, fainting, chest pain or pressure, numbness, or tingling should also be checked immediately.

CREPITUS Another warning sign is crepitus, which is almost any sound emitted by a body part that's not working correctly. Squeaking, grating, or rubbing all qualify; there's even "snowball crepitus," resembling the sound of walking on snow, which is usually a sign of tendinitis (inflammation of the tendon).

When you exercise regularly, you must acknowledge that your capacities do decrease with age. Realize too that an area that's been injured is going to have a lower tolerance for stress.

Myth: **The more exercise the better.**

Fact: **As with most things in life, moderation is important. Extreme or compulsive exercise can lead to injury.**

Some Common Injuries

Under no circumstances do we recommend self-diagnosis of pain and injury. You can suffer concomitant injuries—for example, neuritis while you have muscle strain, while you have a sprain, while you have a bruise, while you have a stress fracture—and it takes a health professional to determine the true mechanism of injury. Nevertheless, there are common injuries you should be able to recognize in order to avoid aggravating them further.

STRAINS   Probably the most common type of injury, strains are damage to the muscle or the muscles' components from stretching, ripping, or tearing of its connective tissue. (Tendinitis, for instance, occurs where the muscle attaches to the bone.) There may not be visible signs of muscle strain, but for the most part it hurts to stretch and contract a muscle that's been strained. Stretching it will increase the temperature and make the pain more tolerable, but the ache will return at rest.

Tennis elbow. Tennis elbow is one of the most common types of strain, usually the result of ballistic maneuvers in racket sports. It appears in the group of muscles known as the forearm extensors. It can be avoided with isometric wrist extensions (pressing the wrist against an immovable object for six to eight seconds). Because it can involve nerve irritation, tendinitis may require injected medicine for treatment.

Plantar fasciitis. Another common strain is plantar fasciitis, a muscle strain relating to the mechanics of the foot. The bowstring supporting the long arch of the foot can be excessively stretched, causing pain when it bears weight. This common injury is worsened by running uphill on your toes, or even bouncing on your toes. Anytime you concentrate force on a small area where it can't dissipate to other joints, undue stress occurs. Untreated, plantar fasciitis can lead to heel spurs, which may require surgery or injected medicine to correct.

Shinsplint syndrome. One of the easiest injuries to get—and one of the least understood—is shinsplint syndrome. Shinsplint syndrome is actually a general term covering half a dozen theories for pain in the lower leg. It can refer to muscle strains, or perhaps irritation of the membrane over the bone. Shinsplints occur when the intensity of activity is suddenly increased before the muscles involved are properly conditioned, and they can usually be prevented by stretching, good flexibility, and proper footwear. Unfortunately, shinsplints can be the precursor to a condition called compartment syndrome. Left untreated, it can eventually cause crippling vascular damage and foot problems.

SPRAINS Also very common, sprains relate to joints as strains relate to muscles. In a sprain, tearing or stretching occurs in the connective tissue of the joints, such as the ligaments. Swelling and even deformity often indicate a sprain.

Treating Injuries with RICE

Sometimes, self-treatment is perfectly acceptable. Treated correctly, minor injuries heal without developing into major problems. You simply need to follow some common tenets regarding the use of heat and cold therapy.

Contrary to what you may believe, heat should never be applied to a new injury. It's tempting to ease the soreness with heat from a bath, water bottle, lamp, or heating pad, but if an injury is swollen, it may indicate internal bleeding and swelling. Increasing heat, just as in warm-ups, brings more blood to the injury, which increases the bleeding and swelling. It may be comfortable, but it's not beneficial.

To treat new injuries—whether strains, sprains, or bruises—use the RICE principle:

Rest   **I**ce   **C**ompression   **E**levation

REST   Rest is a very important part of the healing process. You cannot continue to put undue stress on injured tissue and expect it to heal properly. This may mean completely eliminating a certain activity for a while, or maybe wearing a protective splint and brace to give that particular body part a rest.

ICE   When you apply ice to a body part, it decreases the blood flow to the area via vasoconstriction—the capillaries constrict and their walls become less permeable, allowing less blood to flow into the tissues. Cold therapy makes the battlefield smaller, so to speak, thus reducing the area of injury from lack of oxygen. Ice lowers the metabolic rate so that less oxygen is needed and the proximate area isn't damaged. It is also an anesthetic, numbing pain and reducing muscle spasm.

Myth: Women need special guidelines to exercise safely.

Fact: Common sense applies equally to both sexes. Both women and men need to be careful to prevent injuries.

As with all facets of injury prevention, there are rules to follow with ice: It can, after all, be dangerous if applied incorrectly.

1. Always apply cold with an insulating layer—a towel, plastic bag, or even submersion—but never with a stationary, static application.

2. Ice the injury for twenty minutes, then let it warm for about one hour; then repeat. Another alternative is ice massage—essentially, rubbing ice over the injured body part—but that should be done for no more than twelve minutes at a time.

3. For a significant injury, continue the cycle of twenty minutes of cold treatment and sixty minutes without treatment for twenty-four to thirty-six hours. Only after that period of time is it safe to apply heat, and then as locally as possible; sitting up to your neck in a tub of hot water is not going to help your ankle. Also remember that moist heat works far better than dry heat—a moist hot pack is more therapeutic than an infrared lamp.

4. Finally, avoid balms or ointments that may have a derivation of the word "heat" in their brand name. As skin irritants that only give the sensation of warmth and comfort, they are not true therapeutic heat as they don't increase the blood flow to the area, or its temperature.

COMPRESSION   A compressive or elastic bandage may be helpful in keeping swelling to a minimum. However, it should not be worn so tightly as to completely restrict blood flow.

ELEVATION   Elevate the injured area as often and as high as possible. This also helps decrease swelling. For example, if you injure your ankle, lie on a couch with your ankle propped up on pillows so that it is higher than your heart.

Injury Avoidance Checklist

1. Understand any special conditions your body may have, and exercise appropriately.

2. Include warm-up and cool-down as part of your exercise routine.

3. Make sure your shoes fit properly and your clothes allow evaporation of sweat.

4. Know the difference between pain and discomfort.

5. Don't try to diagnose an injury yourself.

6. Treat minor injuries using the RICE principle: rest, ice, compression (such as elastic bandage), and elevation.

Keeping *Your Back* Healthy

Terrie Heinrich Rizzo, M.A.S.

By investing just a few minutes a day in exercise, you can dramatically decrease your odds of suffering back pain.

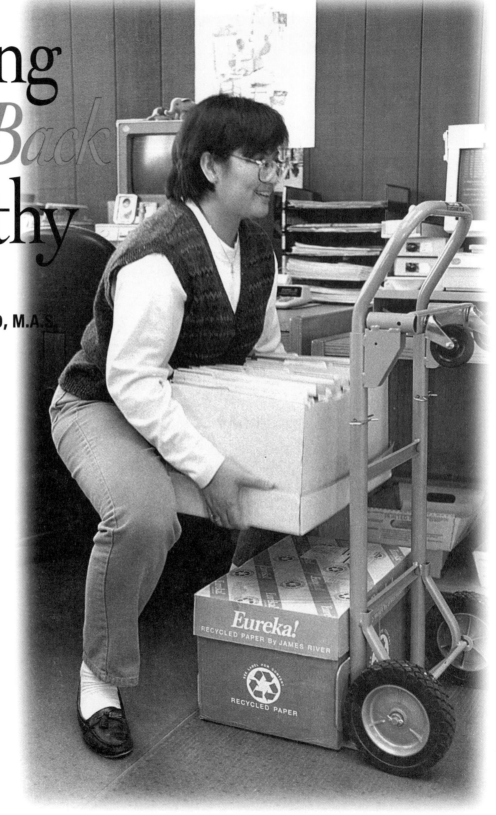

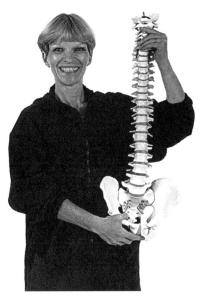

*B*ACK PAIN IS…well, quite a pain. Nearly 80 percent of Americans will suffer from some type of back problem at some point in their lives, and in 30 to 70 percent of these cases, the pain will recur at least once. Of *these*, about 5 percent will go on to develop into a chronic back pain condition. Back pain is the second leading reason for visiting a primary care physician (after the common cold), and it accounts for 25 percent of all days lost from work. If you've ever had a back problem, you know how debilitating even a minor backache can be and how it affects virtually every area of your life.

Although many people attribute back problems to "getting older," back pain and disability surprisingly do *not* get progressively worse with age and do not correspond to the natural age-related changes of spinal disc degeneration. Statistically, incidences of back problems actually peak at around age forty—lack of conditioning, stress, and poor body mechanics are believed to be important factors. Gender is not an issue when it comes to backs: Men and women are equally afflicted by back problems.

Once back pain occurs, recovery usually takes between three days to six weeks. Statistics indicate that 45 percent of back pain episodes disappear within one week, and nearly 80 percent of sufferers have recovered after four weeks. However, for a small but dramatically affected minority of about 5 percent, the acute back pain becomes chronic. Research shows that people who miss work for longer than six months because of low-back pain have only a 50 percent probability of ever returning to work, in great part affected by emotional distress, depression, and adaptation to living with chronic pain.

Terrie Heinrich Rizzo, M.A.S., is Manager of Health and Fitness Education Programs for the Stanford Health Improvement Program. Among her responsibilities are the development and implementation of employee programming at Stanford for office ergonomics and back injury prevention. Her exercise program includes teaching a Healthy Back/Strong Abs exercise class several times each week.

The Healthy Spine

The spine is made up of twenty-four vertebrae, arranged in three curves that form a natural "S" shape:

1. Your head is supported by the seven vertebrae of the cervical spine.

2. Your ribs, which protect the internal organs, are attached to the twelve vertebrae of the thoracic spine.

3. Your lower back, which is the "workhorse" of the spine and the site of most back pain, is composed of the five vertebrae of the lumbar spine; these absorb nearly all torso stress when you sit, stand, or move.

When the cervical curve, thoracic curve, and lumbar curve are properly aligned, you are less vulnerable to injury and pain. "Good posture" means keeping your back curves in balance and aligned, regardless of activity. Other structures support the spine and allow you to move to perform a wide variety of activities:

- *Intervertebral discs* are the tough fibrous and gelatinous "cushions" that separate the vertebrae.

- *Ligaments* connect the bones of the spine to each other and to the pelvic ring, to provide stability while permitting a healthy range of motion.

- Finally, hundreds of *muscles* support the spine and enable you to move in all directions.

Whether severe or mild, back pain clearly is a problem that affects the quality of life for millions. However, most people can decrease the odds dramatically with the investment of just a few minutes daily. How? By *consciously* following a few simple rules of body mechanics and by actively working to maintain a strong, flexible back and supportive muscles.

What Happens to Your Back as You Age?

When we are in our twenties, natural changes begin to occur to the spine that can increase the back's vulnerability. As we age, the intervertebral discs tend to dry out and thin, becoming less resilient and resulting in the vertebrae moving closer together. At the same time, the ligaments that join the vertebrae tend to become looser, permitting a "shimmy" between the bones. The intervertebral foramen, where the nerves of the spinal cord exit, become smaller, permitting a greater chance of pressure on a nerve or nerves (a condition called spinal stenosis). And finally, because of the shimmy caused by looser ligaments, the muscles supporting the back are called on to work harder, which can cause greater muscular tension or tightness.

Although these physical changes in the spine happen at different rates in different people, they are all part of the normal aging process—similar to hair turning gray. Whether these natural changes lead to a back problem for *you* depends a great deal on how you take care of your body. In other words, what you do (or don't do) plays a major role in determining whether "degenerating discs" or other physical changes lead to an aching back. The good news: Much of this is related to lifestyle issues over which *you* have control.

What Causes Back Pain?

The vast majority of back problems are *not* the result of underlying physical diseases. In fact, organic diseases (such as arthritis, osteoporosis, or ankylosing spondylitis) are the cause of back pain in fewer than 20 percent of episodes seen by physicians.

Instead, most trauma to the back is the direct result of *biomechanical* causes—that is, the overloading or stressing of the spinal structures (muscles, vertebrae, joints, ligaments, or intervertebral discs) due to compression, tension, or shearing forces when you move.

- *Compressive* forces push vertebrae and discs together, such as when you lift a heavy weight.

- *Tensile* forces (tension) act on ligaments and muscles, such as when you bend forward in an extreme position.

- *Shearing* forces (twisting) can cause trauma to the vertebrae, discs, or ligaments, for example, when you fall on an icy parking lot, or even just twist to hit a tennis ball or reach the telephone.

Biomechanical stress or overloading occasionally happens during a sudden accident, but it occurs far more commonly during all kinds of everyday movements—lifting a box that's too heavy, twisting to get a tool, or even picking up something as light as a piece of paper. However, while one specific move may be the "culprit" to which you point as the direct cause of your backache, research shows that the underlying lifestyle factors that set up most back problems are stress, poor posture, incorrect body mechanics, and lack of exercise.

Stressing Out Your Back

Stress can be and often is a precursor to back pain, due to the body's automatic responses when faced with a stress-provoking situation. Because the autonomic nervous system cannot differentiate between kinds of stressors, your body's reactions are identical whether you are stressed by being stuck in a traffic jam or being chased by an enraged bull.

This fight-or-flight response, which prepares you for action, is perfectly healthy—provided it is merited in the first place and you can use the energy it creates (as you would when running away from the bull). But when the response is inappropriate (such as getting upset by a situation over which you have no control) or kept up for too long without release, it may start to generate harmful stress and nervous tension.

How does this relate to your back? One of the primary physical reactions in preparation for fight-or-flight is the contraction of the muscles of the entire body—including the

> "No doubt about it: Exercise that strengthens the muscles—especially abdominals—and promotes flexibility will help relieve and prevent back pain."
>
> —Terrie Rizzo

muscles of the back. If your body is frequently or continually under stress, it is easy to see how your back can suffer the consequences.

Coping with stress, then, is essential to a healthy back; learning and practicing effective techniques to manage stress not only will help you cope in general, but also will help relieve or prevent back pain. You either must use up the energy created by the fight-or-flight response, such as with appropriate action or exercise, or learn how to dissipate the response with conscious relaxation. See the chapter Mind + Body: The No-Stress Equation for some suggestions about how you can manage your stress.

Poor Posture

Remember the spine's three natural curves? If you have good posture, those three curves are maintained in place as you perform your daily activities, thus resulting in a minimum of muscular fatigue or wear and tear on your body.

However, poor posture (rounded shoulders, locked knees, slouching, or other exaggerated postures) not only throws your spine's three curves out of alignment, it actually can *accelerate* the aging process of the spine. The negative effects can include abnormal pressure on the discs, stretched ligaments, static muscle loading (holding a muscle in a contracted position), continual muscular fatigue, and, in general, excessive "wearing" of the spine.

If you have poor posture, over time your stronger muscles take over and lead to a muscular imbalance—which in turn leads you to unconsciously adapt by learning to move with the wrong group of muscles. To keep or regain good posture,

Self Test: How's Your Posture?

Many aches and pains that seem to have no specific cause can be attributed to poor posture. As an adult, you may have postural habits that are deeply ingrained due to sore joints and weak muscles, but they can be changed. Take this opportunity to assess your posture accurately, and then work consciously to stand up straight and sit properly.

Use the following guidelines when you assess your posture:

- Wear a minimum of clothing.
- Use a full-length mirror.
- Have someone help you with the side and rear views, or have two mirrors at right angles so you can see yourself in profile. You can also take pictures or videotape yourself.
- Relax and assume your natural, normal posture throughout the tests.

Use the following diagrams to see if your alignment is desirable or imperfect. For each postural problem, a specific remedy is recommended.

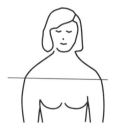 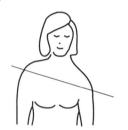

UNEVEN SHOULDERS

This can be caused by carrying a heavy bag on one shoulder. Place your backpack across both shoulders, or change the side you carry your purse on every day.

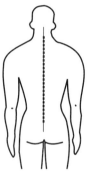 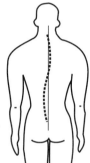

SIDEWAYS CURVATURE OF SPINE

You have a common condition known as scoliosis. An extremely mild sideways curvature may not create a problem during exercise, but an obvious curve should be evaluated by a medical expert.

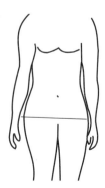 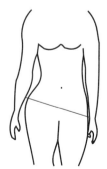

UNEVEN HIPS

If your shoulders and knees are also uneven, you should be evaluated by a medical expert.

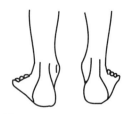 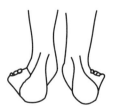

OVERPRONATION

People who suffer from excessive pronation often have a flat-footed appearance. If in doubt, seek the advice of a specialist. You may need to be fitted with custom-made corrective devices that fit inside the shoe and support the foot.

you need to develop a *balance* of flexibility and tone among *all* muscle groups and joints, so that certain groups are not stronger or weaker than others. For most people, this means that an active program of exercises for both strength and flexibility is essential, especially as you age.

Incorrect Body Mechanics

Biomechanically, there are "good" and "bad" ways to perform every kind of daily activity: lifting, bending, pushing, pulling, sitting, standing, even sleeping. Using correct body mechanics enables you to perform the activity efficiently with the least possible stress to your body—for example, bending your knees to reach to the floor for a dropped pencil.

On the other hand, the "bad" way (using incorrect or inefficient movements) increases the risk for everyday wear and tear. Or, even worse, an overload that can become an immediate pain episode—such as bending over from the waist to get the pencil on the floor. Ouch!

Every daily activity that you perform correctly means one less movement that puts you at risk for biomechanical overloading. Paying attention to your body mechanics takes only a few seconds, but it can help you avoid days of pain. *Here are some easy and effective suggestions for maintaining good body mechanics:*

1. *Keep your weight down.* Extra pounds put your back under extra pressure and significantly increase your chance of an injury. Even fifteen to twenty extra pounds force your back to work harder, and put stress on hip and knee joints.

2. *Always use good lifting technique.* Statistically, the num-

How to Lift Anything Without Hurting Your Back

1. Stand as close to the object as possible.

2. Keep your legs shoulder-width apart.

3. Bend both of your knees, keeping your upper body as upright as possible.

4. Bring the object close against your body, then raise up, unbending your knees and keeping your upper body as upright as possible.

5. To place something on the floor, simply reverse the above process.

Back-Friendly Computer Use

It's easy to get so locked into your computer that you sit inches from the screen for hours without moving. This is bad in general, and terrible for your back. Here are some tips for back-friendly computing:

- To help prevent yourself from hunching over, be sure the top of the monitor is roughly level with the top of your forehead.
- Use a document holder to hold source materials in order to keep your head upright.
- Use a footrest if your feet do not comfortably reach the floor when your knees are slightly higher than your hips, and use a lumbar support or any other aids necessary to keep your back supported and hold your body in neutral position.

ber-one immediate cause of back injury is lifting something—even a pencil—incorrectly. Always pay attention to the lifting rules in this chapter.

3. *Push instead of pull, every time you can.* You actually have about twice as much power when you push, and it puts less strain on your back. Try to keep your elbows as close to your body as possible, and your head up.

4. *Don't twist or strain when reaching.* Use a tool or ladder to reach high objects. Keep your entire body facing the object, and bring the object down and in, as close to your body as you can, as you lower it from above.

5. *When sitting, consider your back:* Sit so your lower back and feet are supported, and make sure your knees are level with, or slightly higher than, your hips.

6. *On the telephone:* Use a telephone headset or neck rest to help save your back and neck

7. *Don't sleep on your stomach:* This is the worst sleep position, because it forces the back's natural "S" curves into an arch for hours. Try instead to sleep on your back (with a pillow under your knees) or in the fetal position (with a pillow between your knees). Consider purchasing a "body pillow" to help give all-night support, no matter how you sleep.

Lack of Exercise and Your Back

Several unfortunate things usually happen to muscles and joints that are not worked properly, leading to a general imbalance between loose and tight muscles and between stiff and unstable joints. Research indicates that these imbalances can play a *major* role in affecting your back's ability to withstand the normal effects of both aging and the biomechanical stresses of everyday activities. To put it bluntly, being out of shape virtually guarantees back problems!

MUSCLES   In healthy people, muscles do not relax completely but maintain a slight degree of contraction, referred to as *muscle tone.* When muscles are not exercised regularly—whether the result of disease, improper movements, or plain old inactivity—they lose their tone and do not contract as powerfully as they should: The result is less support for the bony structures of the body.

At the same time, other muscles often become too tight. These muscles also do not contract as powerfully as they should, are weaker, and are more susceptible to injury. Tight muscles can result from several causes:

- Injury (as the muscle spasms to protect itself from further injury).

- Stress (part of the fight-or-flight response).

- When active joint movements are not maintained through daily stretching activities.

- Certain types of physical activities (for example, heavy manual work).

Shoulder Bags and Your Back

Never carry a heavy shoulder bag! The weight of the average shoulder bag forces you into improper posture (one shoulder lower than the other and back twisted out of alignment). If you must carry a shoulder bag, lighten it up. Better yet, use a handbag or light fanny pack. The same principal applies to heavy garment bags. Instead of lugging an overweight bag around the airport, use a portable travel cart or luggage with wheels.

- Certain kinds of exercise (such as weight lifting) also can cause the "musclebound" condition of "tighter" muscles, particularly if stretching exercises are not included to maintain necessary balance.

JOINTS Joints also can be dysfunctional in two ways: by becoming hypermobile (loose and unstable), resulting in too much movement; or by becoming immobile (fixed and stiff), resulting in an overall loss of movement. When a joint has become hypermobile, the ligaments will be loose and the supportive muscles usually become tense and sore in an attempt to compensate for and minimize the excessive movement.

When a joint has become stiff, the ligaments will usually be much tighter than they should be, and muscles lose their flexibility as well. Because the back has many segments, immobility at one joint will often mean compensatory changes producing hypermobility at adjacent joints. Therefore the effects of poor posture, previous injury, stress, or even the natural changes caused by aging (remember the "shimmy"!) can be disastrous, especially if you add lack of exercise to the mix.

The greatest support you can give your back is to build and maintain strong and flexible supporting muscles and joints. And the only way to do that is to exercise properly!

Commonly Asked Questions About Exercise for Backs

Q: *I've been told my back pain was caused by lumbar strain/degenerating discs/facet syndrome/osteoporosis/scoliosis. Should I do back exercises?*

A: For any pain disorder, always get advice from your health care provider before attempting specific exercises. In general, except for serious conditions, once an acute episode is under control, regular exercises can help eliminate or at least minimize back problems.

Lumbar strain. This is back pain that doesn't seem to have any cause. Stretching and toning exercises (and weight loss if overweight) usually are a major help in reducing the symptoms of lumbar strain and in preventing recurrence. Be sure to check with your doctor before you begin.

Degenerative disc disease. This usually occurs in an older age group, as "degenerating discs" are part of the normal aging process. Stretching and toning exercises can help provide maximum muscular support, minimizing weaker bony support.

Facet syndrome. This is a condition of discomfort in the neck caused by weight-bearing on the facet joints (where the vertebrae meet) instead of on the vertebral body and discs. Extending the head backward increases the discomfort. A common cause is poor posture or imbalance of supporting muscles, and can be improved with appropriate regular exercises.

Osteoporosis. Osteoporosis, which also usually occurs in an older age group, is a weakened condition of the bone caused by loss of calcium. It often causes partial collapse of one or more vertebrae. Although osteoporosis is more common in women, it is sometimes found in older men as well. Exercise plays an important role in the *prevention* of osteoporosis, particularly the regular performance of weight-bearing aerobic exercise and strength exercises to maintain muscle mass. Following the onset of the disease, appropriate regular exercise can help provide maximum muscular support and help slow the disease progress.

Scoliosis. This is a sideways curve in the spine. Although scoliosis can be caused by bony changes, much of the effect of the condition can be improved by strengthening and improving the balance of the supporting trunk muscles through exercise.

Q: *Would exercise help a sciatica problem?*

A: Sciatica is a description of pain that "shoots" or localizes in one or both legs and may radiate down to the foot and toes. Sciatica may be accompanied by weakness of muscles, numbness, or diminishment or loss of reflexes. It is usually caused by pressure on a nerve root that supplies one or both legs; this pressure is most commonly caused by a herniated disc, spinal stenosis, or a narrowing of the intervertebral foramen.

Following proper diagnosis and conservative care, exercise can be a major help in the rehabilitative process and in preventing further recurrences. You should have personal advice from your physician concerning appropriate exercises.

Q: *Why does my back feel worse after exercising?*

A: Some discomfort at the beginning of an exercise program is quite normal, particularly if you haven't exercised at all in the recent past. The situation results from the "progressive overload" principle, which in this case means that when an out-of-shape muscle is exercised, some overload can be expected. You can minimize discomfort through following a *gradual* program of exercise that allows the muscles and joints time to adapt to exercising, and by always following recommendations for proper warm-up and cool-down.

Q: *I have a specific problem—degeneration of the L5-S1 disc. What does this mean?*

A: This means that the particular disc has become thinner, narrowing the space between the two vertebrae on either ·side—in this case the disc between the lowest of the five lumbar vertebrae and the first of the five fused tailbone vertebrae (L means lumbar or lower back; S means sacral or tailbone).

Degenerating discs are a normal part of the aging process, and studies suggest that the most common degenerative changes occur in the lower back, in the L4-L5 and L5-S1 discs. Remember that having a specific problem often is not the *total* problem, since muscular and joint imbalances usually contribute to overall discomfort. A regular balanced exercise program helps relieve or prevent pain even when specific problems are present.

Q: *Should I wear a back belt when I exercise or go to work to prevent back problems?*

A: Current research suggests that support belts are not the solution for back problems. Overuse or overreliance on belts can cause sloppy body mechanics and weaken the abdominals by doing the work for them.

We discourage use of a belt during most exercise (for lifting heavy weights, see the chapter Using Your Muscles for Life), and at work or home to prevent back problems—*except* when very heavy weight is to be supported above the waistline in any way, including standing, sitting, or especially bent over. Otherwise, pay attention to proper body mechanics, use good techniques, and develop strong and flexible muscles, particularly abdominals and spinal muscles.

Exercising for a Healthy Back

Although all the exercises included in this book are safe and effective for most people, you should use caution when appropriate. It is not uncommon to experience some soreness or mild back discomfort after beginning a back exercise program, particularly if you have not exercised in the recent past. However, if you continually experience pain while exercising, consult your physician.

For a strong, healthy back, follow an overall program of physical exercise that emphasizes general fitness, aerobic capacity, and the specific conditioning or reconditioning of the muscles that support the spine. Make sure you include stretching, strengthening, and aerobic activity in your workout program.

STRETCHING AND STRENGTHENING   Include exercises to improve both the strength and flexibility of the muscle groups that support the spine. The most common weaknesses and imbalances that contribute to back pain—and which should specifically be addressed through exercise—are the following:

- tight hamstring muscles (need stretching)
- tight mid-back and low-back muscle groups (need stretching)
- tight hip flexor muscles (need stretching)
- weak abdominals (need strengthening)
- weak upper-, mid-, and low-back muscle groups (need strengthening)

WARM-UP AND COOL-DOWN   An adequate warm-up and

cool-down is essential: Always begin exercising with a light warm-up, such as a few minutes of walking or light marching in place, to prepare your body for the work ahead. And always be sure to cool down appropriately following the exercise period.

For specific instructions on how to do stretching and strengthening exercises, see the chapters on Stretching for Flexibility and Using Your Muscles for Life. Here are the rules in short.

For stretching:

- Stretch slowly to your point of tension and hold for at least fifteen to thirty seconds.

- Don't bounce.

- Don't hold a painful position.

- Relax, keep breathing, and concentrate on the area being stretched.

For muscle-strengthening exercises:

- Try to maintain good body alignment at all times.

- Don't try to overdo a movement by moving higher, faster—more is not better!

- Stop and rest if you feel a "burn" or any kind of discomfort.

AEROBIC EXERCISE   Exercises for your back will help improve your overall strength and flexibility, but they will not provide you with the third important component of fitness, aerobic conditioning. You will need to include this in another way to burn calories and strengthen your cardiovascular sys-

Remember!

Before you begin a program of back exercises, remember the following warnings:

- If you have any current or chronic back problems, consult with your physician before attempting any specific exercises.

- Don't perform an exercise if you experience pain.

- Make back exercises part of an overall, balanced program of exercise and everyday adherence to good body mechanics.

tem. In addition, by using good body mechanics as you perform everyday activities, you increase the effectiveness of your exercise program by reducing daily wear and tear and reducing the risk of injury.

Remember: For a strong, healthy back, follow an overall program of physical exercise that emphasizes general fitness, aerobic capacity, and the specific conditioning or reconditioning of the muscles that support the spine. Make sure you include stretching, strengthening, and aerobic activity in your workout.

Exercises to Help Your Back

Among the best exercises for backs are stretching exercises for flexibility and abdominal strengthening exercises (see Stretching for Flexibility and Using Your Muscles for Life for other good exercises). Here are some exercises that are particularly good for backs.

TORSO TWIST FOR LOWER BACK AND HIP ROTATORS *Benefits: stretches lower back, hip, and outer thigh.* Lying on your back and keeping shoulders and back flat, gently lower knees to the right, allowing the left ankle to rest on the right ankle. Gently draw the left knee across the torso toward the right shoulder, and then press the left hip back and down toward the floor until you feel a gentle stretch in the left lower back and buttock/hip. Turn your head toward the opposite (left) side. Be sure to keep both shoulder blades on the floor and shoulders down. Hold fifteen to thirty seconds. Repeat to the other side.

TORSO TWIST FOR LOWER BACK AND HIP ROTATORS

Lying on your back and keeping your shoulders and back flat, gently lower your knees to right, allowing the left ankle to rest on the right ankle.

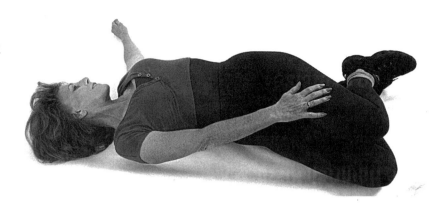

THE PELVIC CLOCK *Benefits: stretches lower back.* Lie on your back with knees bent and feet flat. Imagine the face of a clock resting on your pelvis. First, tilt your pelvis up, flattening the lower back to the floor. This would be a movement to twelve o'clock on the imaginary clock face. Now tilt your pelvis forward. This would be a movement to six o'clock.

Move the hips to opposite numbers on the pelvic clock. For example, move your pelvis back and to the left to the one o'clock position, and then diagonally down and to the right to seven o'clock. Then move from two o'clock to eight o'clock, from three o'clock to nine o'clock, and so on around the clock.

You may find that some numbers are difficult to reach, either because of tightness in certain areas of the lumbar spine or because of lack of control, or for both of these reasons. Go only as far as you comfortably can in each direction, with the goal of eventually achieving equal movement in all clock positions.

Perform all movements slowly and with control. Try not to push with your feet to make the movements. Use only your abdominal and buttock muscles.

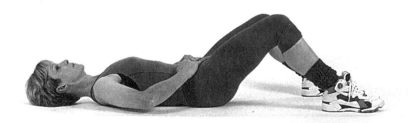

THE PELVIC CLOCK

Tilt your pelvis up to twelve o'clock, flattening the lower back to the floor. Then move your hips to "follow the clock."

KNEE TO CHEST LOWER BACK STRETCH *Benefits: Stretches lower back and hip extensors.* Lie on your back with left leg slightly bent. Grasp right leg behind the thigh. Keeping head on floor, slowly draw right knee up toward chest to facilitate a lumbar and buttock stretch. Hold fifteen to thirty seconds. Repeat with other leg.

KNEE TO CHEST LOWER BACK STRETCH
Grasp right leg behind the thigh and slowly draw right knee up toward chest.

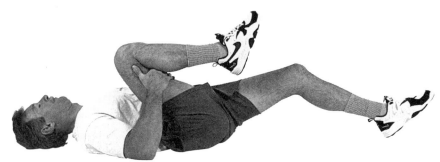

OPPOSITE ARM AND LEG EXTENSIONS *Benefits: Strengthens upper and lower back.* Start on hands and knees, with hands positioned under shoulders and knees under hips. Keep head straight and eyes facing floor. With foot lightly flexed, lift left leg until leg is parallel to floor. Then lift right arm until hand is parallel with floor. Hold ten to thirty seconds. Repeat with opposite side. *Caution: Be sure to keep abdominal muscles tightly contracted. Don't arch your back or let your back, head, or stomach droop.*

OPPOSITE ARM AND LEG EXTENSIONS
With foot lightly flexed, lift left leg until leg is parallel to floor. Then lift right arm until hand is parallel with floor.

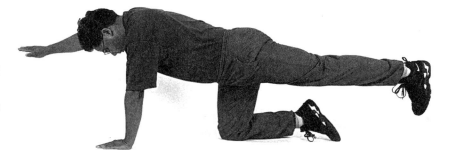

Abdominal Exercises

The most important thing you can do to correctly train your abdominals is to use proper form! To perform abdominal exercises most effectively, it is important to learn good positions that actively stabilize your back and that minimize the involvement of other muscles, particularly your hip flexors and your neck and shoulders. Remember: You are doing these exercises to strengthen your abdominals!

SOME COMMON MISTAKES   Here are some of the more common errors people tend to make when doing abdominal exercises, especially beginning exercisers:

Pulling the neck to perform the movement. To avoid neck pulling, do not lace fingers behind head—instead, lightly support head with fingertips. Also, keep your chin "neutral" by trying to hold an imaginary tennis ball between your chin and chest as you do the entire sequence of the exercise! Try lightly pushing your head *backward* into your hands to take the pressure off your neck.

Throwing the body or using jerking motions. Even if it means you do fewer repetitions, do all motions smoothly, without sudden jerks.

Arching the back. Keep the back stabilized by following the techniques outlined below.

Not lifting your head, neck, and shoulders as one unit. Instead of trying to lift your shoulders, concentrate on *pushing* your rib cage toward your pelvis as you keep your chin neutral—this will cause your entire upper body to move as a unit.

Letting momentum or other muscles do the work, instead of

Abdominal Prescription

1. Try to do at least three different abdominal exercises.

2. For each, beginners should start with three sets of five repetitions, with a stretch between sets. Go slowly—avoid quick, rapid movements.

3. Gradually work up to at least three sets of ten repetitions each.

4. Do these at least three times a week.

5. As your muscular endurance improves, adjust your routine by following the general rule: First, increase the number of reps, then the difficulty. Your muscles should always feel "worked," but not excessively fatigued.

STARTING ABDOMINAL POSITION

This is your active training zone—your feet should be in this position when doing curls and crunches.

actively working the abdominals. Traditional straight-leg sit-ups or even the safer bent-knee position for curls or crunches *do not* actively help stabilize the pelvis and lower back. These positions allow the muscles of the hip flexors and legs to do much of the work, rather than the abdominals that are supposed to be strengthened, or they allow the feet to passively stabilize your back against the floor rather than making your abdominals work to do it. See the photo of a sit-up to avoid in the chapter Don't Hurt Yourself!

FINDING YOUR POSITION   It's important to find your best foot position for abdominal work to actively stabilize your back. To find this position for yourself, start with your legs straight. Try to press your back flat to the floor using only your abdominals. (You will notice that your knees naturally bend as you tilt your pelvis to flatten your back.) Bend your knees and move your feet closer to your buttocks until you can flatten your back using your abs. This is your "active training zone"—your feet should be in this position when doing curls and crunches for greatest effectiveness.

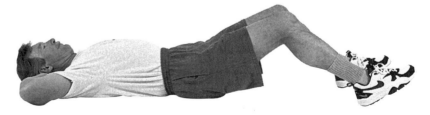

BASIC ABDOMINAL CURL   Start with your knees bent in your active training zone, hands supporting head, elbows out to sides. Slowly lift rib cage to clear shoulder blades off floor. Hold. Slowly lower to starting position.

BASIC ABDOMINAL CURL
Slowly lift rib cage to clear shoulder blades off floor.

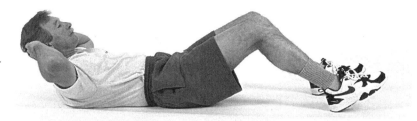

ABDOMINAL TILT AND CURL Start with your knees bent in your active training zone, hands supporting head, elbows out to sides. Contract abdominals to tilt hips. Then lift rib cage to clear shoulder blades off floor. Hold. Lower shoulders. Release pelvis to neutral. *Note: This looks a lot like the Basic Abdominal Curl, but they are two very different exercises. This one is more difficult and works the lower belly.*

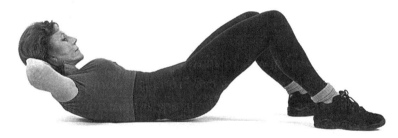

ABDOMINAL TILT AND CURL
With abdominals contracted to tilt hips, lift rib cage to clear shoulder blades off floor.

ROTATION CURL Start in basic curl position and very slightly lift rib cage to raise shoulders. Using right shoulder blade as a pivot on the floor, press left rib cage (not elbow!) toward opposite knee. (It may help you to imagine a magnet on your left shoulder drawing it toward your right knee.) Return to square position without relaxing.

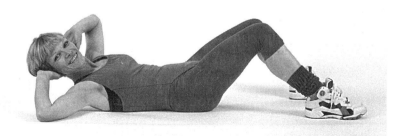

ROTATION CURL
Using right shoulder blade as a pivot on the floor, press left rib cage (not elbow!) toward opposite knee.

REVERSE CURL   Start on your back with elbows to sides and fingertips pointing to ceiling. Raise knees over hips, so that knees and hips are fully extended (bent) and heels close to buttocks. Contract abdominals. Pull abdominals to lift hips slightly off floor. Return knees to starting position. Note: Movement will be small, not large!

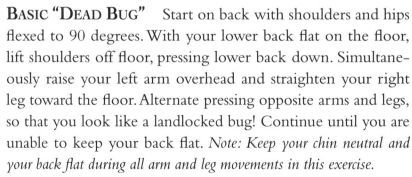

REVERSE CURL
Pull abdominals to lift hips
slightly off floor.

BASIC "DEAD BUG"   Start on back with shoulders and hips flexed to 90 degrees. With your lower back flat on the floor, lift shoulders off floor, pressing lower back down. Simultaneously raise your left arm overhead and straighten your right leg toward the floor. Alternate pressing opposite arms and legs, so that you look like a landlocked bug! Continue until you are unable to keep your back flat. *Note: Keep your chin neutral and your back flat during all arm and leg movements in this exercise.*

"Press and Reach" Variation: Start on back with shoulders and hips flexed to 90 degrees, as in Basic "Dead Bug." Simultaneously *slowly* raise both arms overhead and straighten one leg toward the floor. Return to starting position and repeat, lifting both arms and straightening opposite leg. Continue until you are unable to keep the back flat.

BASIC "DEAD BUG"

Start on back with shoulders and hips flexed to 90 degrees. Simultaneously *slowly* raise one arm overhead and straighten one leg toward the floor.

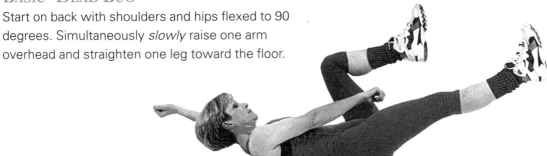

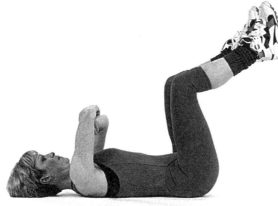

"PRESS AND REACH" VARIATION

Start on back with shoulders and hips flexed to 90 degrees. Extend both arms overhead *slowly* and straighten one leg toward the floor.

RAISED LEG CURLS AND TWISTS   Start by lying on your back close enough to a bench or chair so that your calves are supported. Your knees should be directly over your hips, so that your legs form a 90-degree angle at your knees and hips. Consciously press your lower back to the floor. Lift rib cage to clear shoulders off floor. Hold. Return. Alternately, press rib cage toward opposite knee. Return.

RAISED LEG CURLS AND TWISTS

Consciously press your lower back to the floor. Lift rib cage to clear shoulders off floor.

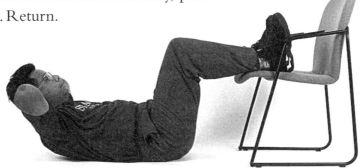

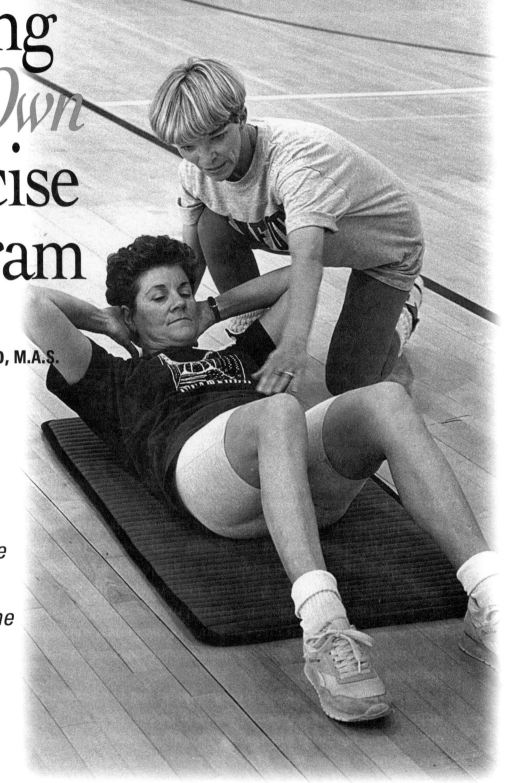

Creating *Your Own* Exercise Program

Terrie Heinrich Rizzo, M.A.S.

If you do exercise that's fun for you, you're one step closer to being able to maintain your exercise plan for the rest of your life!

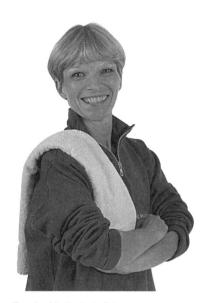

Terrie Heinrich Rizzo, M.A.S., is Manager of Health and Fitness Education Programs for the Stanford Health Improvement Program. She also is Executive Director of Personally Fit/Belgium, which she established in 1981 as one of the first aerobics programs in Europe. A health and fitness educator, she has taught aerobic dancing and body-conditioning classes weekly for over twenty years. She also enjoys dancing and cross-country skiing.

N O ONE KNOWS YOUR EXERCISE needs better than you. In this chapter, you will learn what you can do to create your own personal exercise program and how to maintain it for the rest of your life!

The Four Pillars of Exercise

Here are four important points to remember before you begin: get moving, build up slowly, do it regularly, and maintain your program.

First, get moving. Make a firm commitment to exercise as a regular and natural part of your life, whether you take up new activities or find a more active way to do the things you do now.

Second, build up slowly. If you throw yourself too quickly into a new activity with all of your energy and good intentions, you are likely to burn out or get injured.

- Make sure that it is medically safe for you to start.

- Take time to get fit, so you don't feel uncomfortable during or after the activity.

- Always warm up before you start and cool down after your workout, to help avoid injury.

- Increase the amount of activity you do by no more than 10 percent each week.

Third, do it regularly. Your program will not work if you don't keep it up.

- Get into the habit of regular exercise—at least twenty minutes a day, three times a week.

Myth: It's best to exercise first thing in the morning.

Fact: Any time of day is a good time to exercise—as long as you find a time that's convenient and comfortable for you.

- Include the three basic types of exercise—aerobic, strengthening, and flexibility—as essential parts of your overall fitness program.

- If you find you have a list of excuses for not exercising regularly (such as "I'm too tired" or "I don't have enough time"), see the chapter No Excuses! for help. You will probably find your most cherished excuses exploded there—as well as ways to help you overcome them.

- Try to cross-train—that is, do more than one type of exercise. Cross-training helps prevent boredom and repetition—two of the downfalls of many exercise programs—and reduces the risk of overuse injury.

- Pick the kind of exercise that fits your personal style. For example, do you prefer group or individual activities? Are you a morning "lark" or an evening "owl"? Do you like a regular routine, or do you need more flexibility in scheduling? Your answers will help you determine the fitness activities that best suit your exercise style, and will make it more likely for you to keep it up as a regular part of your life.

- Schedule your exercise in advance—write it down on your calendar, as you would a doctor's appointment. Then treat exercise as a regular part of your schedule that is as important as any other activity. Consider your exercise time as your regular appointment with yourself.

- Consider joining a class or arrange to exercise with a friend. This will make it harder for you to change your mind and skip your workout at the last minute.

Finally, maintain your program. You're only fit so long as you exercise. You will need to find ways to keep up the regular exercise habit. Here are some strategies you might try:

- Set realistic, short-term goals—ones you can actually achieve.

- Promise yourself a reward after three months (or decide to enter a sporting event that is at least three months away, and set that as your goal).

- Tell everyone you know that you have begun an exercise program. They will help hold you to it.

- Be aware that there are predictable drop-out times: after one month, three months, six months, and one year. Gear yourself up to work through these exercise "hazards" by developing a program that you enjoy—and be ready to work yourself through the tough times!

Are You Ready to Begin?

Will you need a medical examination before you start? Probably not. For most people, starting an appropriate exercise program poses no hazard. Almost everybody can safely exercise at a low to moderate level of intensity, following the guidelines outlined in the chapter Get Moving, Keep Moving—Aerobically. However, you might benefit from a medical checkup if any of the follow apply to you:

- If you have a history of heart disease, high blood pressure, lung disease, or disease of the bones or joints that could be made worse by excessive exercise.

Self Test: The Physical Activity Readiness Questionnaire

Physical activity does not pose a problem for most people. The Physical Activity Readiness Questionnaire (PAR-Q) has been designed to identify the small number of adults for whom an increase in physical activity might be inappropriate, or those who should have medical advice concerning the type of activity most suitable for them. If you answer "yes" to any of the questions below, consult with your doctor before starting an exercise program.

1. Has your doctor ever said you have heart trouble? **Yes No**

2. Do you frequently have pains in your chest? **Yes No**

3. Do you often feel faint or have spells of severe dizziness? **Yes No**

4. Has a doctor ever told you that you have a bone or joint problem such as arthritis that has been aggravated by exercise, or might be made worse with exercise? **Yes No**

5. Has a doctor ever said your blood pressure was too high? **Yes No**

6. Are you over age sixty-nine and not accustomed to vigorous exercise? **Yes No**

7. Is there a good physical reason not mentioned here why you should not follow an activity program if you want to? **Yes No**

Source: *British Columbia Medical Journal* 17 (1975): 375-78

- If you are sedentary, over thirty-five, and intend to plunge immediately into exercise that is more vigorous than brisk walking.

- If you are interested in finding out your current level of fitness to use as a benchmark against which to measure future progress.

If you do feel the need to consult with a doctor before you begin, a range of medical advice is available. A simple evaluation might consist of having a conversation with your regular physician. A more complex evaluation, carried out by an exercise specialist, would include evaluations of body composition, flexibility, and blood lipids. It would also include a treadmill or bicycle test to evaluate cardiovascular function and functional capacity.

Most people do not need a special medical evaluation. We recommend that you follow guidelines for regular medical check-ups. Mention your exercise program to your doctor on your next visit, and ask for his or her advice.

In general, any person under sixty-five with no overt heart disease, high blood pressure, or orthopedic condition can start a gradual program of walking, bicycling, or swimming without undue risk. To test your readiness right now, take the "Physical Activity Readiness Questionnaire."

Stretching, Strength, Aerobics: The Total Program

Your exercise program must be complete to give you all the benefits of exercise. And complete means that your overall program must include exercises for flexibility, strength, and cardiovascular health (aerobics).

MAINTAIN YOUR FLEXIBILITY   Flexibility is important for at least three reasons: to prevent injury while exercising, to allow for flowing movement in daily living, and to help prevent lower-back problems.

Remember, it is important to stretch *moderately*, hold the stretch for fifteen to thirty seconds, and *don't bounce*. Although some stretching exercises are specific to the sport or exercise

> "You don't need to hire a personal trainer to create your own exercise plan! Just include stretching, strengthening, and aerobics, and do activities you enjoy."
>
> —Terrie Rizzo

you perform, there are many that are useful in promoting overall flexibility for everyone, no matter what endurance- or strength-building activity you choose. For more details and some effective exercises you can add to your program, see the chapter Stretching for Flexibility.

BUILD AND MAINTAIN YOUR STRENGTH   Much of the time you spend in physical activity probably will be devoted to aerobic exercise, which builds cardiovascular endurance and offers many overall benefits. But it is also important to spend time building strength. Everyone needs good-quality muscles—not just body builders. Unless you conscientiously maintain your strength, it will decline, making routine tasks—and exercise itself—harder to perform. Additionally, maintaining strength and muscle mass is important for many other health reasons (see the chapters Using Your Muscles for Life and You're Never Too Old to Be Fit).

Unless your aerobic exercise includes a strength portion, as do many aerobic dance classes, you will probably need to add strength-building exercises to keep your body's development in balance. For example, if your main exercise is walking or jogging, which uses primarily your leg and lower body muscles, you may want to develop abdominal and arm muscles with curl-ups and push-ups. See the chapter Using Your Muscles for Life for specific suggestions.

AEROBICS FOR HEART HEALTH   If you want a healthy heart, you must do exercise that results in a sustained elevation in metabolic, cardiovascular, and respiratory functions. In the process, the blood must supply oxygen steadily to the exercising muscle for fuel. That's where we get the term "aerobic," meaning "with oxygen."

An aerobic exercise is any activity that you can maintain continuously, is rhythmical, and uses large muscle groups. The most common aerobic activities include: brisk walking, jogging, skating, cycling (at 10 miles per hour), swimming, cross-country skiing, stationary cycling or stepping machines, and aerobic dance. Activities like doubles tennis or golf (if you ride in a cart) are excellent recreational activities, but they're not vigorous enough to enhance cardiovascular endurance; and games like softball, while fun, do not keep you moving continually.

Shaping Your Exercise Plan

Here's how your exercise session should shape up:

1. *A ten-minute warm-up period,* including general movements to warm up the cardiovascular system and stretching exercises to prepare the joints being used.

2. *A twenty- to sixty-minute aerobic period,* for cardiovascular endurance, three to five times per week.

3. *A five- to ten-minute cool-down period,* including further stretching and strengthening exercises.

Additionally, each week you need to do:

4. *A twenty- to thirty-minute strength-training program* that includes all major muscle groups of the upper and lower body. This should be done a minimum of two times per week. This can be combined with your aerobics program; or, if done alternately, be sure to warm up, stretch, and cool down appropriately.

Warm-up and Cool-down

For some, warm-up and cool-down may seem the most boring parts of any exercise program. However, they are very important to prevent injury, to balance muscle development, and to prepare your cardiovascular system for strenuous activity and calm it down afterward.

WARM-UP   In general, your warm-up should follow this pattern:

1. Slow, large movements such as arm circling, arm swinging, and slow walking.

2. Stretches that exercise the muscle groups you will be using in your aerobic portion, as well as stretches for flexibil-

Exercise and Sleep: You Need Both

Of all the components of health and fitness, sleep is the one we most often neglect. Although researchers don't fully understand the mechanisms of the relationship between sleep and exercise, they do know that getting enough of both is essential to health.

Everyone needs between six and nine (or more) hours of sleep daily. Studies show that even short-term lack of sleep can have negative effects on everything from our ability to handle stress to our immune system. Lack of sleep also affects exercise.

According to William Dement, Ph.D., director of the Stanford University Sleep Disorders Clinic and Research Center, "People who get enough sleep are much more energetic, are more positive, have better reaction times, are better able to concentrate on their performance, and are more likely to adhere to a regular exercise program."

Conversely, tired exercisers are more likely to be careless and lack good judgment—for example, they may not stretch properly, or they may overestimate their abilities. Additionally, people who haven't gotten enough sleep lack motivation—which means they're less likely to do today's workout or stick to any long-range exercise program.

Experts feel that exercise enhances sleep.

Aerobic exercisers fall asleep more quickly, experience more slow, deep-wave sleep, and sleep longer than nonexercisers. Here are some recommendations:

1. Don't exercise within three hours of bedtime. It can make you feel "wired" and make sleep difficult.

2. Take sleep seriously. Take your needs seriously and get help with symptoms of chronic sleep problems, especially severe snoring.

3. Learn how much sleep you really need. You'll know you're sleeping the right amount when you wake up rested, alert, and ready for the day every day for a week.

4. Condition yourself for sleep. Deal with stressful problems earlier in the evening, take a warm (not hot) bath to relax, make your bedroom a "no-work" zone—use it only for sleeping and sex.

5. Correct poor sleep habits. Go to bed and get up at the same time every day. Avoid late-evening stimulants that interfere with a good night's sleep—caffeine, alcohol, and nicotine.

6. Use the exercise-sleep relationship to benefit your health. Make sleep a part of your exercise program, and exercise to enhance your lifetime sleep habits.

ity of the neck, shoulders, trunk, hip, hamstring, calves, and Achilles tendon. Remember: Don't bounce; and hold each stretch at a degree of mild tension (before the muscle begins to shake) for approximately fifteen to thirty seconds.

COOL-DOWN During cool-down, walk around for a few minutes until your breathing rate and heart rate are well below the target zone. Do not stop exercise abruptly—this may result in lightheadedness or fainting due to blood pooling in the legs. You might perform another set of stretching while your muscles are still warm. For more information, see the chapter Stretching for Flexibility.

Aerobic Exercise

This is the main part of your exercise session. The activity you choose is up to you, but whatever it is, you should be able to answer "yes" to these three questions:

1. Am I enjoying myself?

2. Am I doing the exercise safely, without risk of damage to my joints, muscles, or heart?

3. Am I exercising at the proper intensity for me?

The first question is key: If you are miserable or are bored, you'll probably quit. Look for an exercise you like, prevent boredom by mixing different types of exercise, and arrange for pleasant company while you work out.

FINDING THE RIGHT DEGREE OF INTENSITY The second and third questions hinge on the intensity with which you exercise. You need a certain degree of intensity to condition the cardiovascular system, producing the overload that leads to physical fitness. You can determine this level of intensity in two ways: (1) the amount of oxygen you are capable of using during exhaustive work (known as your VO_2max) and (2) by the speed that your heart beats.

Myth: Eating protein builds muscles.

Fact: Using muscles builds muscles—be sure to include strength training in your exercise program and eat a balanced diet.

For more about VO$_2$max—which requires a graded exercise test measuring your inspired and expired air—see the chapter Why Exercise Works. For instructions on finding your target heart rate and other self-monitoring techniques, see the chapter Get Moving, Keep Moving—Aerobically.

The easiest—and perhaps best—technique is simply to listen to your body. Let your heart rate and feeling of exertion be your inner coach.

HOW LONG AND HOW MUCH? In addition to a ten-minute warm-up period (and a five- to ten-minute cool-down), the period of aerobic exercise should last at least twenty minutes. As you become fitter, you will benefit by increasing this period to forty or even sixty minutes. The recommended frequency is every other day, up five days a week. On your off days, continue the conditioning process by increasing your routine activity (walking, gardening, cleaning your car or house, and so on).

BURNING CALORIES You can also consider using a system that involves keeping track of how many calories you are burning. This will be of particular interest if you want to lose weight, but it is a useful way for anyone to monitor the amount of exercise they are getting.

The recommended caloric expenditure for beginners (those who have been sedentary for a while) is about 750 calories a week. You can derive this from three twenty-minute periods of activity in the target heart-rate zone; one hour of stretches and strength exercises; and one hour of additional routine activity (such as walking or yard work). If you have reached a high level of fitness, and exercise for longer periods of time, the number of calories can rise to about 3,500 a week.

SELECTING YOUR EXERCISE   Instead of picking one exercise and doing it every day, we suggest that you try to mix two or more types. Your physical development will be better balanced, and you will run less risk of boredom. Refer to the chapter Get Moving, Keep Moving—Aerobically for suggestions. There are some advantages and disadvantages to different types, with some practical suggestions on ways to make the most of each activity.

Keeping It Up

The challenge is not starting a program, but maintaining one for the rest of your life. In fact, the hardest part of exercise for many people may be keeping it up after the first feelings of virtue have worn off. Here are some suggestions:

- Try to come up with some strategies for dealing with these problems before they come up.

- Don't set goals you are unlikely to reach, either in terms of time or effort.

- Plan ahead, but don't set up a schedule so rigid that you can't meet its demands and feel guilty as a result.

- Planning activities one week at a time is helpful.

- Arrange to exercise with someone else—this makes it hard to change your mind at the last minute!

Use the sample exercise planner in this chapter to create —and stick to—your own exercise program. Have fun!

Myth: You can exercise away your cellulite.

Fact: Fat is fat! There is no entity known as "cellulite." The best way to get rid of fat deposits is with sustained, moderate-intensity aerobic dance *and* reduced caloric intake.

Exercise Planner

Dates: _____ to _____

I plan to exercise _____ days a week for _____ minutes a day.

I plan to do the following exercises:

Warm-up: _____
_____

Flexibility: _____
_____

Aerobics: _____
_____

Strength: _____
_____
_____

Other: _____
_____

My goal:
_____
_____

Exercise Record

	SUNDAY	MONDAY	TUESDAY	WEDNESDAY	THURSDAY	FRIDAY	SATURDAY
WEEK 1							
WEEK 2							
WEEK 3							
WEEK 4							
WEEK 5							
WEEK 6							
WEEK 7							
WEEK 8							
WEEK 9							
WEEK 10							
WEEK 11							
WEEK 12							

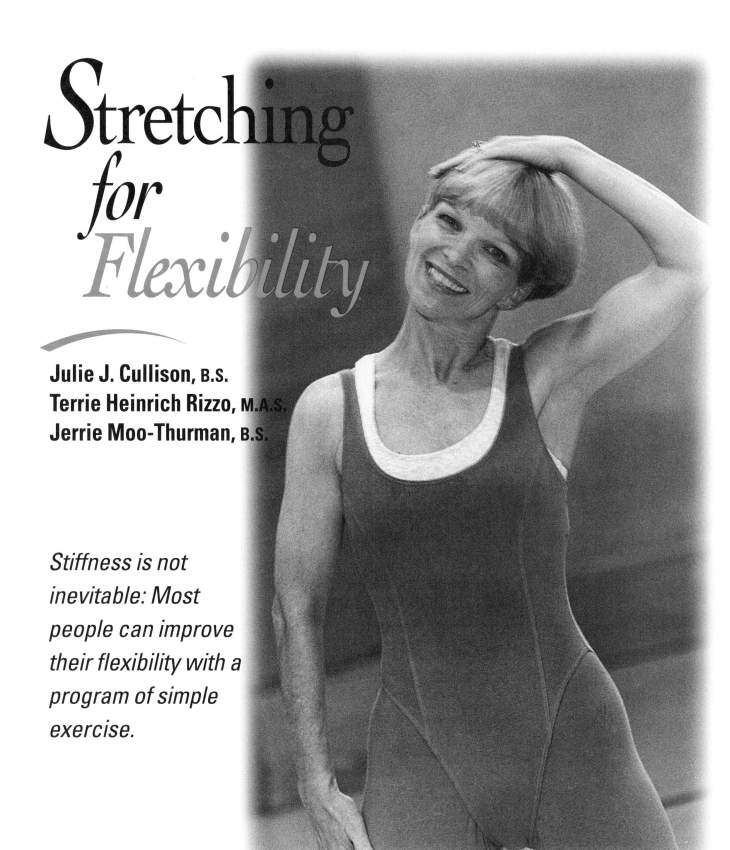

Stretching
for
Flexibility

Julie J. Cullison, B.S.
Terrie Heinrich Rizzo, M.A.S.
Jerrie Moo-Thurman, B.S.

Stiffness is not inevitable: Most people can improve their flexibility with a program of simple exercise.

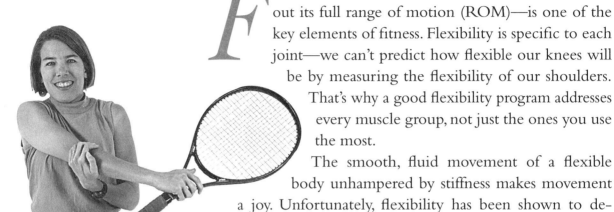

Julie J. Cullison, B.S., Coordinator of the Stanford Health and Fitness Assessment Program, Health Improvement Program. Julie keeps in shape by riding her bike to work and playing tennis. She also likes to go hiking on Bay Area trails.

FLEXIBILITY—THE ABILITY to move a joint throughout its full range of motion (ROM)—is one of the key elements of fitness. Flexibility is specific to each joint—we can't predict how flexible our knees will be by measuring the flexibility of our shoulders. That's why a good flexibility program addresses every muscle group, not just the ones you use the most.

The smooth, fluid movement of a flexible body unhampered by stiffness makes movement a joy. Unfortunately, flexibility has been shown to decrease with age—not necessarily because of biological processes, but as a result of diminishing physical activity that sometimes accompanies aging. This means that stiffness is not an inevitable product of aging: Most people can improve their flexibility with a program of simple exercise designed to increase the elasticity of the muscles, tendons, and ligaments.

A flexibility program is a planned, deliberate, and regular program of exercise that can permanently and progressively increase the range of motion of a joint or a set of joints over a period of time. You should always precede flexibility exercises with a mild set of warm-up exercises that increase body temperature and make the stretching both safer and more productive.

We stretch as a part of a warm-up or cool-down before or immediately after exercise mainly to improve performance and reduce risk of injury in that activity. Warm-up provides the body with a period of adjustment from rest to exercise, and cool-down does the same for the transition from exercise to rest.

How Stretching Helps Your Body

- Reduces muscle tension and makes the body feel more relaxed.
- Helps coordination by allowing freer and easier movement.
- Increases the body's ability to move joints through the full range of motion.
- May help prevent injuries of muscles and tendons.
- Enhances the performance of an activity by signaling the muscles that they are about to be used.
- Develops body awareness by focusing on specific muscles.
- Promotes circulation.
- It feels good!

Although most people think of stretching before they begin a workout, it's even more important afterward. Tissue temperatures are highest immediately after the main part of a workout, so stretching at the conclusion of the workout may keep muscles from tightening up quickly and may help decrease muscle soreness, particularly for people who are not regular exercisers.

Three Types of Stretching

You may have thought that stretching is just stretching, but in fact there are three basic types: static, ballistic, and proprioceptive neuromuscular facilitation (PNF), as explained in the chapter Why Exercise Works. Let's take a brief review of each type.

STATIC STRETCHING   Static stretching is the preferred type because it may result in less muscle soreness, and there is less chance that you will stretch beyond the limits of the muscle tissue. In this type of exercise, you gradually stretch through a muscle's complete range of motion, slowly lengthening the muscle until you feel resistance or the beginning of discomfort. When you reach this point, you hold the position for fifteen to

Terrie Heinrich Rizzo, M.A.S., is Manager of Health and Fitness Education Programs for the Stanford Health Improvement Program and Executive Director of Personally Fit/Belgium. A health and fitness educator, she has taught aerobic dancing and body-conditioning classes weekly for over twenty years. She also enjoys dancing and cross-country skiing.

Jerrie Moo-Thurman, B.S., is Coordinator of Fitness Programs for the Stanford Health Improvement Program and an exercise physiologist with over fifteen years of experience in exercise instruction, health education, and wellness program coordination. She has conducted aerobics training programs in Japan, Mexico, and throughout the United States, and has trained aerobics instructors in college and private training programs. She enjoys dancing, swimming, skiing, and playing sports and games with her husband and two children.

> "Stretching is the most overlooked component of a balanced program. But it's critical to feeling good, preventing injuries, and maintaining lifelong flexibility." —Terrie Rizzo

thirty seconds and repeat the exercise two or three times. Static stretching has been found to be effective in increasing ROM, but is generally more effective in maintaining ROM.

BALLISTIC STRETCHING   Ballistic stretching involves dynamic movements that may be bouncy or jerky. If momentum becomes too great, the actual movement may exceed joint ROM and result in a sprained ligament or tendon. Not surprisingly, ballistic stretching is not recommended.

Each time you stretch a muscle, the opposite muscle relaxes to permit lengthening. In a fast, jerky movement—such as bouncing to touch your toes—the opposite muscle may resist lengthening by contracting as a protective mechanism against overstretching. This can lead to injury because the elastic limits of the muscle may be exceeded.

Myth: Stretching is the best way to start an exercise session.

Fact: Stretching cold muscles actually increases the risk of injury. Always warm up with gentle exercise first—before stretching.

PNF   Proprioceptive neuromuscular facilitation (PNF) requires two people to work together. It is a more complex method of stretching than the first two, but it can be the most effective. Let's look at how one variation, contract-relax (CR), works to exercise the hamstrings and quadriceps. (In this case, we call the hamstrings the *antagonist* muscle group, and the quadriceps the *agonist* muscle group.)

First, the partner moves the exerciser's leg to an end point of ROM and holds it at least ten seconds. This is a passive stretch. After the passive stretch, the exerciser contracts the quadriceps muscle for six to ten seconds. This is followed by another passive stretch of the hamstrings, and then the process is repeated.

Another variation is called contract-relax agonist-contract (CRAC). This technique has been found to have the greatest

Safe and Effective Stretching

1. Warm up for a few minutes before you start stretching by walking, slow jogging, or another gentle exercise.

2. Perform stretches daily, if possible.

3. An optimal session should last ten to twenty minutes, holding each stretch fifteen to thirty seconds to maintain flexibility. To increase flexibility significantly, hold each stretch for one to two minutes.

4. Stretch before you exercise or begin playing a sport to warm up muscles and help prevent muscle strain and perhaps injury.

5. Stretch the specific muscles required for your sport or activity as well as a general stretch of major muscle groups.

6. Move slowly from stretch to stretch.

7. Stretching should be gradual and relaxed. Don't bounce.

8. Minimize the movement of other body parts by focusing on the muscles you want to stretch.

9. Stop if your feel any pain. Any discomfort should be mild and brief at worst.

10. Remember to breathe during a stretch.

11. Perform each stretch at least twice.

12. Stretch after every workout to help prevent muscles from tightening up.

improvements in ROM than either contract-relax or static stretching. The partner moves the exerciser's leg to an end point of ROM, and the exerciser contracts the hamstrings (the antagonists) for six seconds against resistance supplied by the partner. Then the exerciser contracts the agonist (quadriceps) muscle. This is followed by a passive stretch of the hamstrings.

PNF can be effective, but it has several limitations:

• It requires two people working together.

• Without adequate knowledge of the technique, injury can result.

• It produces more pain and muscle stiffness then the other methods.

• It takes more time.

Stretching for General Flexibility

The rest of this chapter contains some simple but effective stretches that are safe to do every day. When you stretch, follow this routine:

Self-Test: How Flexible Are You?

Here are a few simple moves you can do to measure your flexibility. To prepare:

- Dress lightly and comfortably.

- Ideally, another person should assist you. If you are alone, use a mirror to help you see your body positions.

- As you go through the positions, stretch until mildly uncomfortable, but don't force to pain.

- Check the diagrams to see if you meet the suggested flexibility.

Lower back: Lying on your back, pull both knees toward chest. *Goal:* Your knees should touch your chest.

Back of thighs: Lying on your back, lift one leg, keeping the other leg flat on the floor, without bending either knee. *Goal:* Raised leg should reach a vertical position.

Front of thighs: Lying on your stomach with knees together, gently pull your heel toward your buttocks. Repeat with other heel. *Goal:* Heel should comfortably touch buttocks.

Shoulders: Standing, reach one hand backward and up to opposite shoulder blade. Repeat with other hand. *Goal:* Hand should touch bottom of shoulder blade.

1. Before you stretch—whether you are stretching as part of your pre-activity warm-up or for increasing your flexibility—*always* warm up with several minutes of rhythmic, overall body movement such as marching in place, step touches, heel steps, or knee lifts.

2. *Then add* upper-body warm-up work:

- *Shoulder shrugs:* Bring shoulders up, elevating shoulder blades, then lower.

- *Shoulder rolls:* Bring shoulders up, then pull back and down, then around.

- *Backstroke:* Leading with thumb, alternate lifting arms up and back, then around in a circular motion.

3. *Then move on* to your stretches. Standing stretch exercises are especially good for use before engaging in an aerobic or strengthening activity. Floor stretches are good for general flexibility and for cool-down. Whatever stretch you're working on, you should hold all movements for fifteen to thirty seconds. When appropriate, be sure to stretch both right and left sides of the body. When you do standing stretches, be sure

to keep your knees "soft" or slightly bent—don't lock your knees—to minimize back and knee strain.

Remember: Take it easy, take it slow, stop if you feel pain, and don't bounce! Also, if you have neck or spine problems, check with your doctor.

NECK STRETCH (can also be done seated) *Benefits: Stretches neck and upper shoulders.* Tilt head to right, keeping shoulders down. Place right hand on left side of head and gently pull head toward right shoulder. Hold for fifteen to thirty seconds, then do other side. *Caution: Do not drop your head back.*

OVERHEAD SHOULDER EXTENSOR STRETCH (can also be done seated) *Benefits: Stretches shoulders and upper back.* Raise both arms overhead, grasp hands, and gently pull back. Be sure to keep shoulders down and elbows close to ears. Hold for fifteen to thirty seconds.

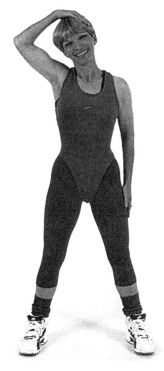

NECK STRETCH
Place right hand on left side of head and gently pull head toward right shoulder.

OVERHEAD SHOULDER EXTENSOR STRETCH
Raise both arms overhead, grasp hands, and gently pull back.

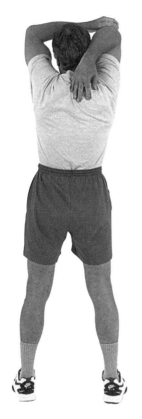

TRICEPS AND SHOULDER STRETCH (can also be done seated) *Benefits: Stretches back of arm and shoulders.* Point right elbow overhead next to ear; with left hand, gently pull elbow so that hand rests on spine, to stretch back of arm and shoulder. Hold fifteen to thirty seconds. Repeat with other arm.

TRICEPS AND SHOULDER STRETCH
Point right elbow overhead next to ear; with left hand, gently pull elbow toward head.

SHOULDER AND UPPER BACK STRETCH (can also be done seated) *Benefits: Stretches back of shoulders and upper back.* Bring right arm across chest; with left hand, gently pull arm across to stretch upper shoulder and back. Hold fifteen to thirty seconds. Repeat with other arm.

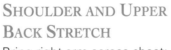

SHOULDER AND UPPER BACK STRETCH
Bring right arm across chest; with left hand, gently pull arm.

CHEST AND FRONT SHOULDER STRETCH (can also be done seated) *Benefits: Opens chest and shoulders.* Clasp hands behind back; turn shoulders around, then press hands down; gently elevate hands one to two inches. Hold fifteen to thirty seconds.

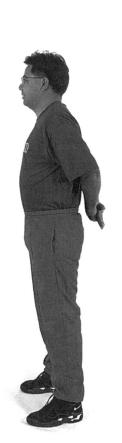

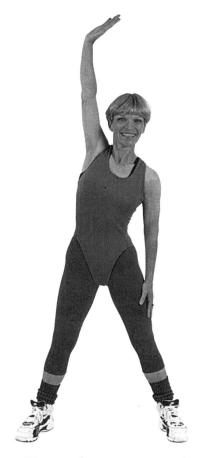

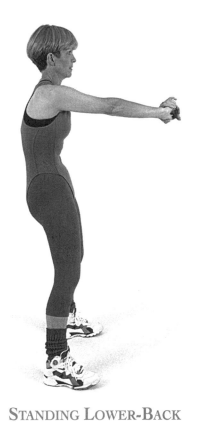

CHEST AND FRONT SHOULDER STRETCH
Gently elevate clasped hands one to two inches.

TORSO STRETCH
Reach hand up, pressing palm toward ceiling.

STANDING LOWER-BACK STRETCH
Round the lower back by tucking the pelvis forward and using the abdominal muscles to produce a low-back tilt.

TORSO STRETCH *Benefits: Stretches sides and torso.* Support left hand on thigh and reach right hand up and over left shoulder, pressing palm toward ceiling, to stretch right side. Keep your hip in! Hold fifteen to thirty seconds. Repeat with other side.

STANDING LOWER-BACK STRETCH *Benefits: Stretches mid- and lower back.* Grasp hands and push forward in front of chest to round upper back. Then round the lower back by tucking the pelvis forward and using the abdominal muscles to produce a low-back tilt. Hold fifteen to thirty seconds.

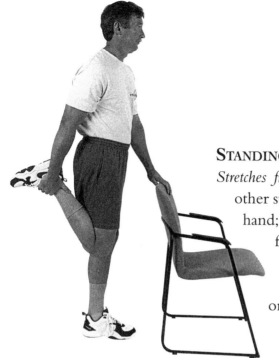

STANDING QUADRICEPS/HIP FLEXORS STRETCH *Benefits: Stretches front of hip and thigh.* Placing hand against wall or other stationary object, grasp right ankle or foot with right hand; gently pull heel toward buttocks, then tuck pelvis forward. Be sure to keep knee close to bottom knee. Caution: Do not arch back or lift knee out to side when doing this stretch. Hold fifteen to thirty seconds. Repeat with other leg.

STANDING QUADRICEPS/ HIP FLEXORS STRETCH
Gently pull heel toward buttocks, then tuck pelvis forward.

STANDING HAMSTRING STRETCH

Benefits: Stretches back of upper leg. Extend left leg forward with foot lightly flexed, then bend right knee and lean slightly forward from hips, using hands for support. Keep knee of extended leg slightly bent, and maintain neutral spine. Caution: Do not round your back or keep forward leg rigid. Hold fifteen to thirty seconds. Repeat with other leg.

STANDING HAMSTRING STRETCH
Extend left leg forward with foot lightly flexed, then bend right knee and lean slightly forward from hips, using hands for support.

STANDING UPPER-CALF STRETCH

Shift body weight forward by bending left knee, keeping right heel on floor, to stretch calf.

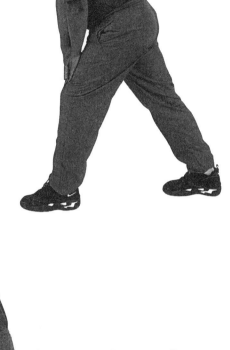

STANDING UPPER-CALF STRETCH *Benefits: Stretches upper calf.* Step forward with left foot, keeping feet parallel to each other. Shift body weight forward by bending left knee, keeping right heel on floor, to stretch calf. Hold fifteen to thirty seconds. Repeat with other leg.

STANDING LOWER-CALF STRETCH *Benefits: Stretches lower calf.* Keeping weight over hips, step slightly forward with right foot, keeping right heel down. Then bend both knees, and tuck pelvis forward to stretch the lower calf. Hold fifteen to thirty seconds. Repeat with other leg.

SEATED HAMSTRING STRETCH *Benefits: Stretches back of upper leg.* Sit on floor with left leg extended and right knee bent to chest. Keeping chest to knee by grasping leg with your hands, and bending from hips, slowly slide right leg forward until a gentle stretch is felt in the back of the left leg. Hold fifteen to thirty seconds. Repeat with other leg.

STANDING LOWER-CALF STRETCH

Bend both knees, and tuck pelvis forward to stretch the lower calf.

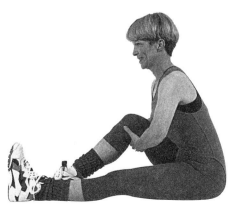

SEATED HAMSTRING STRETCH

Keep chest to knee by grasping leg with your hands, bend from hips, and slowly slide right leg forward.

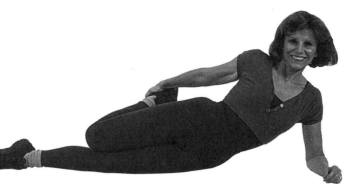

SIDE-LYING QUADRICEPS STRETCH

Grasp right ankle or foot with right hand, and gently pull

SIDE-LYING QUADRICEPS STRETCH   *Benefits: Stretches front of upper thigh.* Lying on left side, grasp right ankle or foot with right hand, and gently pull leg back to feel a gentle stretch in front of thigh. Caution: Be sure to keep knees, hips, and shoulders in alignment. Do not pull knee too far back or arch back. Hold fifteen to thirty seconds. Repeat with other leg.

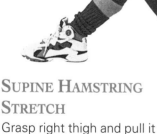

SUPINE HAMSTRING STRETCH   *Benefits: Stretches back of upper leg.* Lying on back with left knee bent, grasp right thigh and pull it gently toward chest until stretch is felt in the back of the thigh. Be sure to keep right knee slightly bent and foot flexed. Hold fifteen to thirty seconds. Repeat with other leg.

SUPINE HAMSTRING STRETCH

Grasp right thigh and pull it gently toward chest.

WHOLE-BODY STRETCH *Benefits: Stretches and elongates entire body.* Lie supine and reach arms overhead and legs forward away from body. Contract abdominals to protect lower back, and *stretch.* Hold fifteen to thirty seconds.

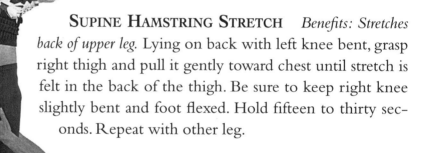

WHOLE-BODY STRETCH

Lie supine and reach arms overhead and legs forward away from body.

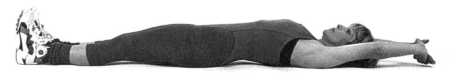

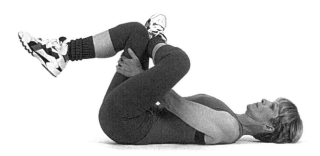

OUTER THIGH AND HIP STRETCH
Grasp thigh with hands and gently pull knee forward until stretch is felt in opposite thigh and hip.

OUTER THIGH AND HIP STRETCH   *Benefits: Stretches outer thigh and hip.* Cross left ankle over right knee; then raise right knee up over hip. Grasp right thigh with hands and gently pull knee forward until stretch is felt in left thigh and hip. Be sure to press lower back to floor to stabilize. Hold fifteen to thirty seconds. Repeat with other leg.

TORSO TWIST FOR LOWER BACK AND HIP ROTATORS
Benefits: Stretches lower back, hip, and outer thigh. See the chapter Keeping Your Back Healthy for this exercise.

SEATED INNER THIGH BUTTERFLY STRETCH   *Benefits: Stretches inner thighs and groin.* Place soles of feet together with heels close to the groin. Grasp ankles lightly with hands, and lean forward while keeping back straight. Then gently press elbows out against the inner thighs. Hold fifteen to thirty seconds.

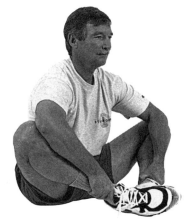

SEATED INNER THIGH BUTTERFLY STRETCH
Gently press elbows out against the inner thighs.

LOWER BACK BASKET STRETCH   *Benefits: Stretches lower back and hip extensors.* Lying on back, grasp both legs behind the thighs, keeping your head in neutral position on the floor. Press your lower back to the floor, and then gently lift buttocks slightly up for a lumbar stretch. Hold fifteen to thirty seconds.

LOWER BACK BASKET STRETCH
Press your lower back to the floor, and then gently lift buttocks slightly up for a lumbar stretch.

Find Time to Stretch

No time to stretch? Think again! Don't limit your stretching to your program. You can stretch during your daily activities without taking any extra time at all.

- *While talking on the phone*: quadriceps stretch, neck stretch, calf stretch

- *While watching television:* inner-thigh stretch, lumbar stretch, hamstrings stretch, chest/shoulders stretch

- *While sitting on an airplane:* neck stretch, triceps/shoulders stretch

- *While working at your desk:* neck stretch, triceps/shoulders stretch, calf stretch, quadriceps stretch

- *While waiting for the light to change*: neck stretch, triceps/shoulders stretch

KNEELING HIP AND GROIN STRETCH *Benefits: Stretches hip flexors, quadriceps, and groin.* Start in kneeling position, with right knee directly over right ankle, keeping body weight over knee. Slowly slide left leg back until you feel a stretch in your left hip and upper thigh. Be sure to keep upper body straight—don't slump over knee! Hold fifteen to thirty seconds. Repeat with other leg. *Note: The weight on your bent leg should be above the kneecap. If your knee is uncomfortable, use a mat or towel to cushion. This stretch is especially beneficial for sedentary people.*

KNEELING HIP AND GROIN STRETCH
Slowly slide left leg back until you feel a stretch in your left hip and upper thigh. Keep your upper body straight.

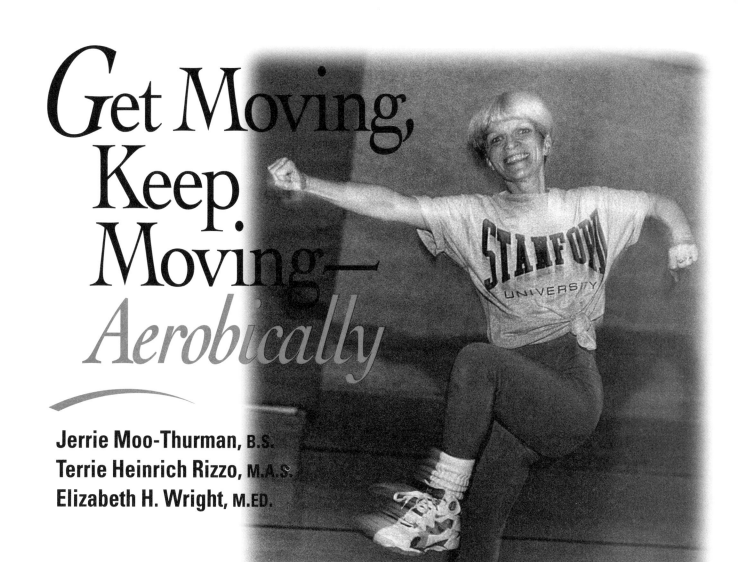

Get Moving, Keep Moving— *Aerobically*

Jerrie Moo-Thurman, B.S.
Terrie Heinrich Rizzo, M.A.S.
Elizabeth H. Wright, M.ED.

The keys to getting results from any aerobic activity are to be consistent and to choose an activity you enjoy doing.

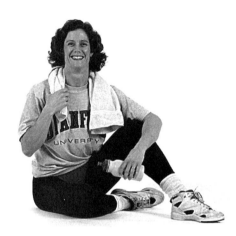

Jerrie Moo-Thurman, B.S., is Coordinator of Fitness Programs for the Stanford Health Improvement Program and an exercise physiologist with over fifteen years of experience in exercise instruction, health education, and wellness program coordination. She has conducted aerobics training programs in Japan, Mexico, and throughout the United States, and has trained aerobics instructors in college and private training programs. She enjoys dancing, swimming, skiing, and playing sports and games with her husband and two children.

WHY DO AEROBIC EXERCISE? Actually, why *wouldn't* anyone do aerobic exercise? As you know from previous chapters of this book, research shows that regular aerobic exercise improves your health and enhances your quality of life in so many ways that the necessary few minutes per week are well worth it!

Benefits to your musculoskeletel system:

1. Improved body composition—body fat is decreased and lean body mass is increased

2. Improved muscular endurance

3. Stronger ligaments and tendons—help prevent injury

4. Strengthened bones—from weight-bearing aerobic activities (those during which you come down on your feet)

Benefits to your cardiorespiratory system:

1. Increased functional capacity of the heart—cardiac output and stroke volume

2. Increased oxygen consumption capabilities—the amount of oxygen that will be used by the muscles to produce energy increases

3. Lowered resting, exercising, and recovery heart rates

4. Possibly decreased blood pressure

5. Improved breathing capacity

6. Improved capacity to sweat more efficiently—conditioned people sweat earlier and more to release body heat

Benefits to your metabolism:

1. Improved blood glucose regulation—helps prevent or regulate diabetes

2. Increased HDL cholesterol levels in the blood—HDL clears "sticky" plaque from artery walls and thus is known as the "good" cholesterol

3. Decreased triglycerides (fatty acids)

4. Promotion of fat loss—by stimulating release of fat to be burned by working muscles

5. Increased caloric expenditure during exercise and for a period of time following exercise

Benefits to your psychological well-being:

1. Improved ability to deal with stress

2. Improved confidence, self-esteem, and a better self-image

3. Improved ability to fall asleep quickly and have better REM or "restful" sleep

4. Increased feeling of well-being and simply "feeling good"

Every single one of these benefits of aerobic exercise has been well-documented by research. Here's how you can make them a reality.

Your Aerobic Exercise Plan

Finding the right aerobic plan to meet your needs and interests doesn't have to be a guessing game. You should ease into an aerobic plan, based on research-based recommended guide-

Elizabeth H. Wright, M.ED., is an exercise physiologist and health educator for the Stanford Health Improvement Program. She is co-ordinator of HIP Off-Site Programs and of the Health and Fitness curriculum of the Stanford Executive Program. Nationally recognized as an accomplished equestrian, she also enjoys participating in triathlons, downhill skiing, and windsurfing. Elizabeth is a certified fitness instructor and has taught movement, aerobics, and conditioning for over eleven years.

Terrie Heinrich Rizzo, M.A.S., is Manager of Health and Fitness Education Programs for the Stanford Health Improvement Program. She also is Executive Director of Personally Fit/ Belgium, which she established in 1981 as one of the first aerobics programs in Europe. She has been a certified aerobic dance instructor for over twenty years, and teaches five aerobics classes weekly. She also gets daily aerobic exercise walking her Airedale.

lines. Use the following guidelines as you plan to fit aerobic exercise into your life.

THE WARM-UP   Always warm up before *any* aerobic exercise. Shinsplints and pulled muscles often are the result of plunging in without a gradual warm-up to raise the temperature of muscles and joints, increase circulation, and improve muscle and joint flexibility.

Here's a good analogy to describe what happens inside your body: Think of your muscles as needing energy to do work just like a fire needs wood to burn. To start the fire, you need paper, kindling wood, and logs. The first to catch fire is the paper, which ignites the kindling for a short period of time, and eventually the logs burn to keep the fire going for hours.

It's the same with aerobic activity. You need to start off with about five to ten minutes of easy all-body movements and flexibility stretches to ignite your body's first energy-producing mechanisms and prepare it to move into the sustained aerobic phase.

Like paper and kindling, the warm-up is crucial to building your body's fire. Examples of all-body warm-ups are slow walking before a more vigorous aerobic walk, slow dancing before moving to faster music, or pedaling the bicycle at a slower speed and with little resistance before you go on to a more energetic ride.

THE COOL-DOWN   A short five- to ten-minute cool-down period after you have finished your vigorous activity is also important. It enables your body to gradually return to a resting state. The cool-down gives your heart a chance to slow down gradually; it gives your body the time to lose some of the heat you generated during exercise; and it gives your muscles the opportunity to relax and stretch out.

To cool down, simply continue your aerobic exercise in slower motion for three to five minutes. For example, after a brisk walk, cool down with a gradual stroll. End a bicycle ride with slow, easy pedaling. Slow down swimming strokes to an easy glide.

Be sure to follow with flexibility exercises. Not only does research indicate that cool-down stretching is an important way to help improve overall flexibility (since your muscles and joints are warm and less stiff than at other times), gentle cool-down stretching also helps reduce muscle soreness that sometimes follows vigorous activity. Be sure to stretch the muscles you have worked, especially hamstring, quadriceps, and calf muscles. For more details, see the chapter Stretching for Flexibility.

THE AEROBIC WORKOUT For maximum cardiovascular benefits, nothing takes the place of aerobic exercise performed at your target heart rate. This means moderate to vigorous exercise performed for a sustained period of time. (However, recent research has shown that many general health benefits also can result with less strenuous activity.)

The types of activity that are considered aerobic exercise include walking at a moderate to vigorous pace, hiking, jogging or running, stationary or outdoor biking, swimming, water exercise, stationary or outdoor rowing, cross-country skiing or ski-machine, stair climber, circuit or interval training, skating, step aerobics, and dance-exercise aerobics.

Myth: The best way to burn fat is to exercise intensely.

Fact: Regular exercise of moderate intensity sustained for longer periods of time is the best way to increase the amount of fat the body burns.

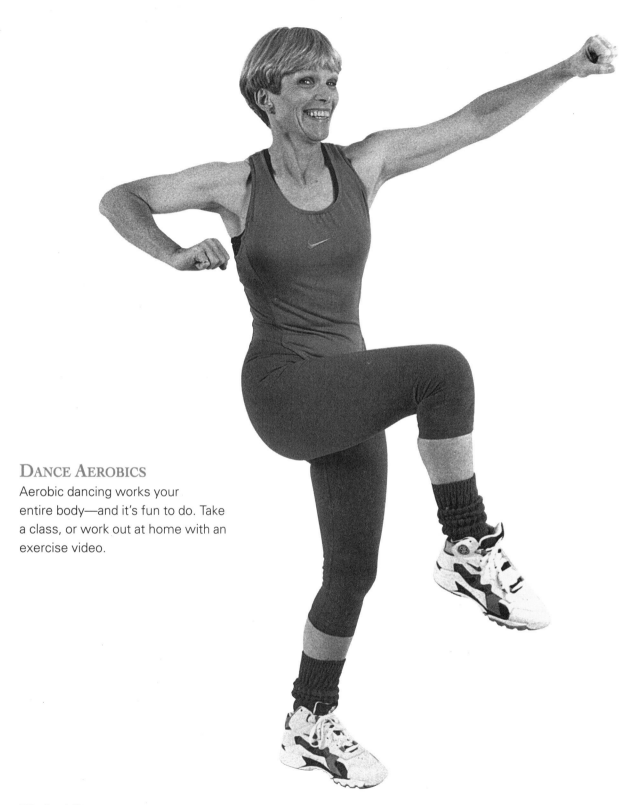

DANCE AEROBICS

Aerobic dancing works your entire body—and it's fun to do. Take a class, or work out at home with an exercise video.

Staying FITT: How Much? How Long? How Hard?

The American College of Sports Medicine recommends the following FITT guidelines for aerobic exercise:

F = Frequency: The frequency of your aerobic activity should be three to five days per week in order to increase cardiovascular endurance. If you have been sedentary, you may benefit from a minimum of two to three days per week. For anyone, participating in more than five exercise sessions per week may not result in appreciable additional benefit and may increase the risk of injury.

I = Intensity: The intensity of the aerobic activity must be between 70 percent and 85 percent of maximal heart rate (slightly less for previously sedentary people). Subjective tests may also be used to estimate aerobic exercise intensity, although these are less quantifiable.

T = Time: The time you spend doing the aerobic activity must be a minimum of fifteen minutes, with an upper limit of sixty minutes.

T = Type: The type of activity you do must be continuous, and must use large muscle groups while doing activities that move the body through a full range of motion.

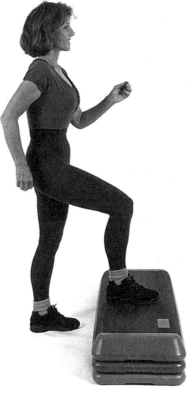

STEP AEROBICS

All you need for step aerobics is a step—buy an inexpensive plastic step, or use a stair at home. Proper Step height depends on individual level of skill, fitness, experience, muscular strength, and predisposition to knee-related problems. Always keep your knee bent at less than a 90-degree angle when stepping onto the platform, and keep your body aligned as shown.

The key to getting results from any aerobic activity is to be consistent. Make a commitment to yourself to get regular aerobic exercise to improve your overall level of physical fitness. As mentioned throughout this book, one of the important factors in being consistent is to pick an activity or activities that you enjoy. If you don't enjoy the activity, you probably won't keep with it for very long. (Research shows that other factors that might affect your consistency are the convenience of the location where the activity will be done, scheduling a regular time of the day that you will do the activity, having a person or a group of people to exercise with, and feeling good after each aerobic activity.)

To ensure that you feel good after every aerobic activity, you will need to pace yourself. This means to modify the moves and the intensity of the activity to your present fitness level. You may also need to be realistic in your exercise pace if you are recovering from an injury, coming back to exercise after a long absence, or if you are not feeling "up to par" that day. You can modify most aerobic activities by moving at a slower pace, or by reducing the resistance against which you have to work. For example, a person just starting a walking program should walk at a moderate pace on a flat surface instead of walking at a fast pace up a hill. Stay within your limits, and don't push yourself to do more than you can comfortably do that day.

When exercising aerobically, you should feel your heart rate and breathing rate increased enough to meet the demands of the exercise, but you should not be out of breath or lightheaded. (These are signals that you're exercising too vigorously and you need to slow down.) To make sure that you are not overworking or underworking during aerobic activity, it is important to pace yourself and to periodically monitor your intensity during the workout.

Monitoring Your Aerobic Exercise Intensity

Monitoring exercise intensity throughout your aerobic activity is a good idea for both new and continuing aerobic exercisers. If you are a new exerciser, you will learn how much or how little exercise you need in order to exercise at the recommended intensity. If you are a continuing exerciser, you will be able to see improvement in cardiovascular functioning when you notice a reduction in heart rate at a given intensity, or when you can perform more work at the same heart rate.

Monitoring also helps you adjust the intensity of your exercise (either harder or not so hard) so that you are exercising within your training zone. The self-monitoring techniques that are easily learned are heart-rate measurement, the Borg Scale Rating of Perceived Exertion, and the Talk Test.

HEART-RATE MEASUREMENT   Heart rate is a reliable indicator of aerobic exercise intensity as long as it is used by healthy adults with normal heart rate responses to exercise, and that it is done correctly. People with certain medical conditions (such as pregnancy), or who take medications that regulate heart rate, will not get an accurate measurement of their exercise intensity with this method. The method you use to take your pulse can also affect the reliability of the measurement.

HOW TO TAKE YOUR PULSE   The most common sites where a pulse can be located are at the wrist (radial artery), at the neck (carotid artery), at the chest (apical pulse), and at the temples (temporal pulse). The preferred location to find your pulse when exercising is the radial artery at the wrist.

    The Radial Pulse To locate the radial pulse, lay the wrist of one arm (palm facing up) in the palm of the other hand. Wrap the fingers of the bottom hand around the wrist of the top hand. The fingers should fall into place on the top of the wrist resting in a soft area in between the radial bone and the flexor muscle tendon.

    The Carotid Pulse If you cannot easily locate your radial pulse, then move to one of the other pulse-monitoring sites. If you are taking the carotid pulse at the neck, be careful to apply gentle pressure and don't massage the side of the neck

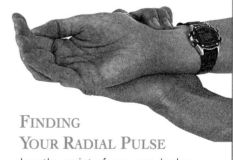

FINDING YOUR RADIAL PULSE
Lay the wrist of one arm (palm facing up) in the palm of the other hand. Wrap the fingers of the bottom hand around the wrist of the top hand.

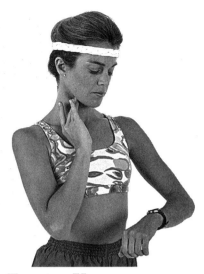

FINDING YOUR CAROTID PULSE

Be careful—use two or three fingers, apply gentle pressure, and don't massage the side of your neck.

1. Use the soft pads of two or three fingers to feel the pulse. Do not use your thumb, which has its own pulse and will obstruct the counting of the actual pulse.

2. Locate the pulse quickly and start counting immediately, preferably within five seconds after slowing down to take the pulse.

3. Count the pulse for ten seconds. The ten-second pulse count is more accurate than the six-second count and is therefore preferred. Starting the count with the number zero is preferred, although starting with one is not incorrect. Consistency in using zero or one is the most important factor in remaining accurate.

trying to find the pulse. (The vagus nerve is near the carotid artery; when stimulated by pressure or massage, it causes the heart rate to slow down and an inaccurate pulse is counted!)

HOW TO FIND YOUR TARGET HEART RATE ZONE There are two methods for estimating what your target heart rate range for aerobic exercise should be: the estimated heart rate intensity chart and the personalized target zone.

The EHRC is an easy—but less personalized—way to determine your target heart rate zone because it is based only on age. The Personalized Target Zone better estimates your true target heart rate zone because both your age and your resting heart rate are factored into the equation.

SIGNS AND SYMPTOMS OF OVEREXERCISING Watch for these signs and symptoms of overexercising both during and after exercise. They indicate the need for you to decrease the intensity, duration, or frequency of exercise.

Symptoms of overexercising during exercise:
- profuse sweating
- very red face
- breathlessness
- inability to keep up with the exercise routine
- facial expression signifying distress
- tightness in the chest
- skin pales or becomes very red
- lack of motivation or listlessness

Self-Test: Finding Your Personalized Target Zone

Here's how you can calculate your personal target zone:

1. To find your maximum heart rate, subtract your age from 220. For example:

220 - 45 = 175 beats per minute

During aerobic exercise, your heart rate should be kept below this number.

2. Now multiply that number by 70 percent and 85 percent to find your target heart rate zone. For example:

175 x 0.70 = 122.5 and 175 x 0.85 = 148.75.

Rounding the numbers, your target one-minute range during aerobic exercise would be between 122 and 149 beats per minute.

3. To find your quick ten-second count, divide your target heart range numbers by six. For example:

122 ÷ 6 = 20 beats per ten seconds

149 ÷ 6 = 25 beats per ten seconds

During exercise, slow slightly (try to keep your feet moving) and immediately count your pulse for ten seconds (this is more accurate than a six-second count). Your number should be within your quick ten-second-count range.

- confusion or disorientation
- nausea
- dizziness
- excessive heart rate

Symptoms of overexercising after exercise:

- sleeping difficulties
- joint soreness or pain
- loss of appetite
- elevated heart rate (over 120 beats per minute) five minutes after stopping exercise

Self-Test: Borg Scale Rating of Perceived Exertion (RPE)

The RPE scale allows you to rate your own exercise effort by using a scale of 6 to 20, which corresponds to exercise as feeling very, very light to very, very hard. For example, if you stated that the intensity of the exercise felt like it was somewhat hard, the corresponding number to this subjective measurement is 14.

This is a good subjective test for beginning exercisers, who often find RPE useful to help develop a sense of how their body feels when exercising within their target heart rate zone. It is also good for people who cannot use heart rate charts, such as pregnant women and those taking medications that alter heart rate.

- 6–7: very, very light
- 8–9: very light
- 10–11: fairly light
- 12–13: somewhat hard
- 14–15: hard
- 16–17: very hard
- 18–20: very, very hard

Symptoms of overtraining: Watch for these signs and symptoms of overtraining. They indicate the need to modify the intensity, duration, or frequency of your exercise.

- loss of body weight when loss is not attempted or desired
- faster than normal pulse in the morning
- unexplained bruising
- restless sleep or insomnia
- reduced capacity to do everyday work
- persistent soreness of the muscles
- persistent joint pain
- decreased appetite
- fatigue that doesn't subside

What Kind of Aerobic Exercise Should I Do?

By now, you probably know that aerobic exercise is not limited to jogging. In fact, you can choose from a wide variety of activities. It's best to have more than one aerobic activity to prevent boredom and to make sure you exercise your entire body. Choose things that are safe, available, and—most important—fun. Don't be afraid to choose different activities as your fitness level improves.

WALKING OR HIKING

Advantages: Walking is easy, inexpensive, and portable. It accommodates a variety of fitness levels and can be social.

Disadvantages: Walking may not be demanding enough for fit individuals unless difficulty of terrain or intensity is increased.

Special considerations: Good shoes are a must. Especially good choice for older people, and those who have been sedentary, are obese, or have joint problems. Hiking on uneven ground increases risk of falling.

RUNNING

Advantages: Running is easy, inexpensive, and can be done both outdoors and indoors. On a treadmill, computerized feedback is possible.

Disadvantages: Higher impact or higher intensities may increase risk of injury; running may aggravate some knee conditions.

Self-Test: The Talk Test

The talk test is an easy test of exercise intensity to be used in conjunction with the heart rate and/or RPE measurement. When you are doing an activity, begin singing your favorite song:

- If you can easily sing every verse, you need to speed up and work harder to make the activity aerobic.

- If you can't get the first line completed without huffing and puffing, you need to slow down.

- If you can sing in short bursts and are breathing deeply but comfortably, this is your aerobic training zone.

If singing isn't for you, do the test by reciting a poem or talking to your exercise buddy.

Special considerations: Good shoes are a must. Intensity and balance are a concern for pregnant women, older people, and those who are obese. Pregnant women must follow their physician's guidelines.

BIKING: OUTDOOR OR STATIONARY

Advantages: Biking can be done indoors or outdoors; it accommodates a variety of fitness levels; it does not put weight on hips, knees, or feet. A wide variety of workout levels are possible with stationary bikes; possible computerized feedback both indoors and outdoors.

Disadvantages: Biking requires equipment, and may aggravate some knee problems. Outdoor biking carries the risk of falls and traffic hazards; stationary biking can be boring.

Special considerations: Biking appeals to a variety of fitness levels. The risk of falling and safety hazards with outdoor biking are a concern for pregnant women, older adults, and the visually or hearing impaired. The bike needs to be properly sized and adjusted. Helmets are essential for outdoor biking.

SWIMMING

Advantages: Swimming can be done indoors or outdoors; it can accommodate a variety of fitness levels; and it does not put weight on any joints.

Disadvantages: Swimming requires skill; chemicals can be irritating to eyes.

Special considerations: Swimming is excellent for almost all people and fitness levels, especially those with joint problems, back problems, or asthma. Caution: You need to swim continuously following FITT guidelines to achieve aerobic benefits.

Myth: You should drink commercial thirst-quenchers and take salt tablets to replace the vital minerals and sodium lost through heavy sweating.

Fact: Nothing is better than water before, during, and after exercise. Salt tablets are not recommended for most physically active people—too much salt puts a burden on the kidneys.

WATER EXERCISE/AQUAEROBICS: SHALLOW WATER

Advantages: Water exercise is social; it offers variety and fun; and can accommodate a variety of fitness levels. Classes often include strengthening and flexibility exercises. Water is an excellent medium for range-of-motion exercises.

Disadvantages: Water exercise requires skill and safety awareness.

Special considerations: This is an excellent mode for all ages and fitness levels.

Possible problems: See swimming (above).

WATER EXERCISE/AQUAEROBICS: DEEP WATER

Same as above. Recommended for those able to swim. Requires flotation device/equipment.

DANCE-EXERCISE AEROBICS

Advantages: Aerobic dance is social and offers variety and fun. It combines creative movement with music, and can accommodate a variety of fitness levels. Classes often include strengthening and flexibility exercises; many types of classes are available to accommodate different needs.

Disadvantages: Aerobic dance requires skill; high-impact classes/higher intensity may risk injury; may aggravate some knee/joint problems if not modified.

Special considerations: Good shoes are a must. With modifications, dance aerobics can accommodate a variety of fitness levels; all moves should be modified to low for deconditioned or older people. Pregnant women should follow their physician's guidelines.

STEP AEROBICS

Advantages: Step aerobics is social and offers variety and fun. It can accommodate a variety of fitness levels by changing bench height.

Disadvantages: There is potential for overuse injuries if step aerobics is used exclusively. It may aggravate some knee conditions. Balance may be of concern for some people.

Special considerations: Good shoes are a must. Beginners must start on a low bench. It is fine for pregnant women, older adults, and obese people, with modifications.

STEP-CLIMBER (MACHINE)

Advantages: A wide variety of work levels is possible; computerized feedback is available.

Disadvantages: Users tend to "lean" on handrails. The lowest levels may be too demanding for those who are out of condition. It may aggravate some knee conditions; can be boring.

Special considerations: Intensity and balance may be of concern for pregnant women and older adults. Pregnant women should follow their physician's guidelines; with modifications, it can accommodate a variety of fitness levels.

CIRCUIT TRAINING: USING WEIGHTS/DUMBBELLS

Advantages: Circuit training combines weighted work with rhythmic aerobics; can offer variety and fun; can be social.

Disadvantages: It requires orientation and education for using free weights/dumbbells.

Special considerations: With modifications, it can accommodate a variety of fitness levels.

*"*Aerobics is at the heart of a balanced exercise program—it's essential to many important health issues. And you definitely don't have to run marathons to be aerobic!*"* —Terrie Rizzo

CIRCUIT TRAINING: USING WEIGHT MACHINES

Advantages: Circuit training with weight machines offer the potential for some greater strength development; can offer variety and fun; can be social.

Disadvantages: It requires equipment, and orientation and education to the equipment. In the home, equipment is specialized and takes up space.

Special considerations: Easy modifications can be made to accommodate older, obese, pregnant, and out-of-condition individuals; pregnant women should follow their physician's guidelines.

INTERVAL TRAINING

Advantages: Interval training is excellent for higher fitness levels; it accomplishes more work in a given time frame.

Disadvantages: Higher intensity may increase risk for injury; may aggravate knee/joint problems.

Special considerations: Know your fitness level and limitations.

CROSS-COUNTRY SKIING (ALSO SKI-TRACK MACHINES)

Advantages: Uses upper and lower body for complete all-body, high-intensity workout; low-impact; can accommodate a variety of fitness levels; outdoor skiing can be social and fun.

Disadvantages: Requires equipment; indoor equipment can take up space; indoor machine can be boring; requires special skill.

Special considerations: With modifications, can accommodate a variety of fitness levels; balance and falling (outdoors) a consideration for pregnant women and people with special needs.

Possible Problems and How to Solve Them

No matter how careful you are, it's always possible to injure yourself while exercising. The following are some common problems that exercisers encounter, and ways to avoid them or make them go away. To learn what you can do to avoid injury, read the chapter Don't Hurt Yourself!

SHIN PAIN/CALF CRAMPS If you have pain around your shins (shinsplints) or cramps in your calves, you may not be spending enough time warming up and cooling down. Be sure footwear is correct, and keep feet and toes relaxed, especially when walking. "Too much, too soon" also contributes to these problems, so be sure to increase intensity and frequency gradually. When walking, running, or dancing, watch for excessive "pushing off" using toes. Since dehydration also causes leg cramps, make sure you maintain fluid intake while exercising.

SORE KNEES/SORE ANKLES If you have sore knees or ankles, you may be moving too fast or with too much impact, putting stress on joints. Reduce impact if possible. To slow your speed and keep your heart rate up, try doing more work with your arms. Also include knee- and ankle-strengthening exercises in your overall program.

NECK/UPPER BACK DISCOMFORT To reduce neck and upper-back discomfort, maintain good posture. Be sure to keep your shoulders relaxed and your chin up. Be sure biking or floor exercises do not cause excessive head flexion or extension. Include stretches for your upper back in your warm-up.

If you have back problems, be aware that certain activities or exercises put you at higher risk because of significant twisting or torqueing motions. These include golf, tennis or racquetball, weight lifting, downhill skiing, and interval training. Substitute less risky activities if necessary. Swimming and water exercise are especially recommended for people with back problems.

BICYCLE-RELATED PROBLEMS Incorrect bike size, seat height, or handlebars may cause a variety of physical problems, especially knee or neck pain. Experiment with different kinds of bike styles or handlebars to find the style that minimizes neck extension.

Here's how to find your proper seat height: Sit on the seat with your heel on the pedal; your knee should be nearly straight when your leg extends to the bottom of the pedal stroke.

SWIMMING/WATER EXERCISE PROBLEMS If chemicals irritate your eyes, wear goggles. Goggles protect your eyes and allow you to keep them open while swimming. If you are sensitive to cold or have Raynaud's syndrome, wear a pair of disposable latex surgical gloves (available at most pharmacies) to insulate your hands.

Using Your *Muscles* for Life

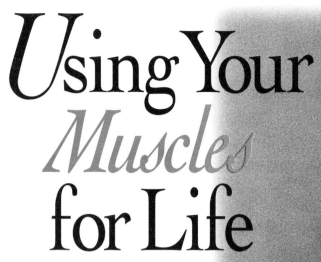

David Krantz, B.S.
Elizabeth H. Wright, M.ED.
Terrie Heinrich Rizzo, M.A.S.
Jerrie Moo-Thurman, B.S.

Recent research shows that people of all ages—that is, every man and woman past puberty—can improve muscle strength and tone.

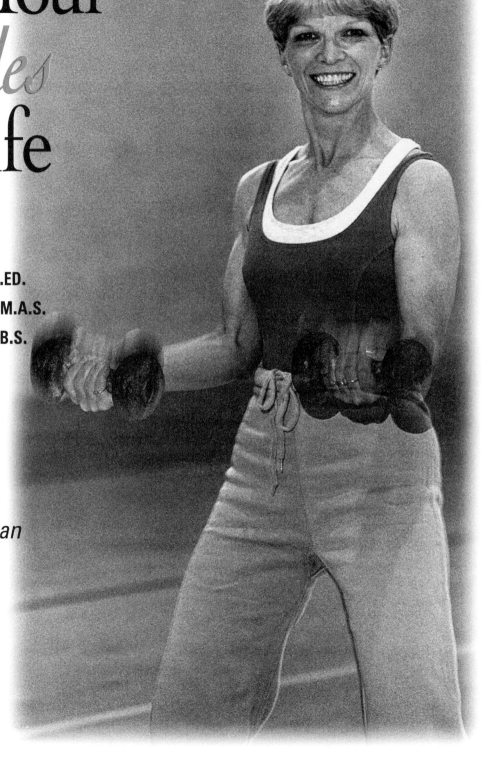

W HETHER YOUR GOALS ARE building, shaping, or just maintaining muscle tone or bone density, virtually everyone—men and women, children and seniors, athletes and beginners—can benefit from this form of exercise:

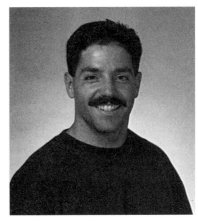

David Krantz, B.S., exercise physiologist and former back program and weight-training specialist with the Stanford Health Improvement Program, is currently pursuing a master's degree in physical therapy. He regularly weight trains, bikes, and runs.

- Your joints may become more stable due to a thickening and strengthening that occurs with strength training, as well as strengthening of the muscles that support certain joints.

- Increased muscle strength means greater physical power, not only during sports, but in all of your daily activities.

- Increased muscular strength may decrease your chances of injury during aerobic exercises that can batter the joints—such has running or high-impact aerobic dancing.

- Women who strength train or perform weight-bearing exercise—especially starting before menopause—may have a decreased severity of osteoporosis because this kind of exercise may build bone density.

You're Never Too Old

Recent research shows that people of all ages—that is, every man and woman past puberty—can improve muscle strength and tone. Our muscle mass and strength tends to peak naturally in our early twenties and decline after about age forty to forty-five. Typically, by about age sixty-five, strength declines by about 20 percent. The great news is that, with exercise, *you can reverse this decline*—even if you are ninety.

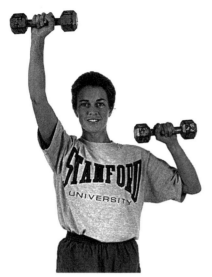

Elizabeth H. Wright, M.ED., is an exercise physiologist and health educator for the Stanford Health Improvement Program. She is coordinator of HIP Off-Site Programs and the Health and Fitness curriculum of the Stanford Executive Program. Nationally recognized as an accomplished equestrian, she also enjoys participating in triathlons, downhill skiing, and windsurfing. Elizabeth is a certified fitness instructor and has taught movement, aerobics, and conditioning for over eleven years.

Some Definitions

applied resistance training: exercise that involves using any form of resistance

barbell: a long weight that must be held in both hands

body building: a sport focused on enlarging and shaping your muscles

circuit training: exercise that involves changing quickly from one exercise station to another

dumbbell: a hand-held weight

muscular endurance: the ability to perform repeated muscular contraction

muscular strength: the force a muscle produces in one effort

repetition: the act of bringing a resistance up, then down

resistance: the hindrance to motion that a weight, rubber tube, or compressed fluid provides

resistive exercise: strength training

set: a group of repetitions

weight: an iron implement for lifting

weight training: resistive exercise that involves lifting any kind of weights

Although younger adults tend to have about twice the ability to gain muscular fitness, improvements can occur at the same rate of increase in previously sedentary individuals whether you are sixty-five or younger. The percent of change is the same for beginners across the board, so you have no excuses for not enjoying strength training, regardless of your age or sex.

Strength training doesn't mean becoming a weight lifter or a body builder. It means doing exercise that provides resistance to muscles to make them stronger—and that's a good idea for everyone. Through strength training, you'll build muscular strength and endurance:

- *Muscle strength* is the ability to lift as heavy a weight as possible one or few times. The more tension you can develop within a muscle during exercise training, the stronger it will tend to rebuild.

- *Muscle endurance* is the ability to lift a weight many times. For endurance or aerobic activities, you will want to exercise for greater muscular endurance rather than strength.

It's a fact that a person who is out of shape will show gains faster than a more fit individual. It's almost as if Mother Nature is trying to encourage the unfit to start exercising. However, the greater fitness you achieve, the more slowly the results will be gained. Improvements happen quite rapidly if you are a beginner, and less so with greater fitness, *but they will happen.*

Before You Lift a Weight, Read This

If you are new to strength training, welcome! Although this should be an important part of your exercise program, you run the risk of injury if you plunge in without a thought to doing it right the first time. In short, before your pick up a weight, you should be aware of a few things before your pick up a weight.

The human body needs time to adapt to a strength-training routine. In fact, the first week or so is a crucial time to be sure to progress slowly. During time, if you feel that you are *not* lifting enough weight, that is the *perfect* amount.

The methods explained here are general guidelines to help keep exercise safe and efficient for most people most of the time. It is impossible to eliminate all sources of injury all of the time, so use due caution.

Terrie Heinrich Rizzo, M.A.S., is Manager of Health and Fitness Education Programs for the Stanford Health Improvement Program. She also is Executive Director of Personally Fit/Belgium, which she established in 1981 as one of the first aerobics programs in Europe. She has taught aerobic dancing and body-conditioning classes for over twenty years.

Jerrie Moo-Thurman, B.S., is Coordinator of Fitness Programs for the Stanford Health Improvement Program and an exercise physiologist with over fifteen years of experience in exercise instruction, health education, and wellness program coordination. She has conducted aerobics training programs in Japan, Mexico, and throughout the United States, and has trained aerobics instructors in college and private training programs. She enjoys dancing, swimming, skiing, and playing sports and games with her husband and two children.

Starting Safely

If you feel that your body is not ready for strength training for any reason, talk to your physician. If you have any of the following risk factors, it is extremely advisable that you see your physician before beginning any strength training program:

- any cardiovascular disease including chest pains at rest or exertion
- family history of coronary heart disease before age 55
- high cholesterol, generally 240 or above
- abnormal EKG, or cardiac arrhythmias
- heavy smoking
- chronic hypertension
- extreme obesity

- any chronic muscular or joint problem or injury, past or present
- within 3 months postpartum or currently pregnant
- recent surgery
- arthritis
- diabetes
- asthma
- years of complete inactivity

Use the following recommendations to prevent injury and ensure a safe and satisfying strength-training routine. Please don't begin until you've read this entire chapter.

DON'T FORGET THE WARM-UP A proper warm-up is essential to preventing injury because it prepares the body for the task at hand. Warming up for strength training has three separate goals:

1. To deliver plenty of fresh, nutrient-rich blood to the areas to be exercised.

2. To warm the muscles. Your muscles actually contract and stretch better after they are somewhat warm.

3. To lubricate the joints, readying them to withstand the extreme forces about to be imparted to them.

If you intend to lift very heavy resistance, perform a few light repetitions before attempting heavy resistance. Without a good warm-up, you may feel a grinding sensation in your joints—and this is *not good*. If this happens, stop the exercise and take more time to warm up further.

WHY STRETCH?   Perhaps you are familiar with the idea that all athletes who lift weights are muscle-bound. This mistaken belief probably came from early weight-training athletes who utterly failed to stretch and possibly failed to exercise through the entire range of motion.

Not stretching can cause muscle-boundness—that is, lack of muscular flexibility. Weight-training athletes are especially susceptible to this because, as the body builds greater and greater muscle tissue, an accompanying state of very slight muscle contraction, or muscle tone, remains. If you have ever felt the relaxed arm of a weight trainer, that hard solid feeling is called muscle tone. Without stretching, this tone can work against you and shorten your muscles, thereby decreasing your flexibility. Clearly, a good stretching routine should be included in any well-rounded exercise regimen.

KEEP IT LIGHT TO LEARN   One of the major pitfalls that newcomers experience is not taking the time to learn proper exercise technique. In order to learn proper form and avoid injury, you should use lighter weights. As an analogy, imagine the difficulty of learning handwriting if pencils weighed ten pounds! During the first week or so, go easy on yourself. Start light and work up.

INTENSITY   Intensity, or amount of effort, can be varied by many factors, including the number of repetitions and sets, the overall amount of weight lifted, and the amount of rest between sets. If you are only interested in strength training as a general means of exercise with no specific goals, you can vary the intensity of your exercise as you see fit.

Generally, the higher the intensity you put into strength training, the greater and faster the results will come. But you need to remember that the higher the intensity, the more likely you may injure yourself or become sore.

LISTEN TO YOUR BODY   The ability to find your proper exercise intensity and guide yourself through a routine by "how you feel" will come only with experience. It takes time to master, but now is a good time to start.

You cannot use heart rate to gauge intensity because strength training causes the heart to pump faster and slower at different times. This variable nature of heart rate responses can make the use of a target heart rate chart very misleading. Furthermore, heart rate alone cannot give feedback on such problems as joint pain. Therefore, while strength training, you will need to rate your perceived exertion based on an overall sense or feeling, not on heart rate. For instructions, see the Borg Scale Rating of Perceived Exertion in the chapter Get Moving, Keep Moving—Aerobically.

HOW MUCH IS ENOUGH?   To maintain minimal muscle strength and endurance, the American College of Sports Medicine recommends a *minimum* of eight to twelve repetitions of eight to ten exercises, at a moderate intensity, two days a week. You'll get greater overall gains with more days per week, sets, and resistance. For example, training two days a week may elicit only 75 percent of the gains that a three-day-per-week program would.

Exercise sessions that last more than sixty minutes tend to have a very high drop-out rate, so we recommend you work

Myth: Muscle will change to fat when you stop exercising.

Fact: Muscles can lose their tone and get flabby, but they can't turn to fat.

for one hour or less per session. Although some programs may elicit greater gains in muscular strength or endurance, most programs will develop both to some degree. Although the amount of rest between sets is largely determined by your goals, you can generally estimate the proper amount of rest by allowing enough time for your muscles to partially recover between sets.

REBUILDING TIME   How much rest or rebuilding time do you need to create strength? After exercise, your fatigued muscles will need a period of rest of approximately one to two days to rebuild stronger. If you are new to fitness or are lifting very heavy weights, you may need the full two days, but as you become more fit, you may need somewhat less time to recuperate. As a general rule, *each muscle* that you train should be rested at least one to two days before being exercised further.

OVERTRAINING   If you sacrifice the one to two days of rest that your body needs to rebuild, this could lead to a progressive weakness of the body instead of progressive gains. This phenomenon, called overtraining, is very much like a nightmare where you try to run harder but only run slower.

Overtraining is extremely difficult to achieve on a three-day-per-week program, but don't consider yourself immune to it. If you are chronically sore or getting weaker, rest: You may

A Word About Lifting Belts

Lifting belts can be purchased at most sporting goods stores in either 6-inch width for general weight training or 4-inch width for competitive weight lifting, as in the Olympics. Either width will do fine for our purposes, but the 6-inch belt may offer a little more support.

The belt is meant to augment the body's own spinal support structures by externally enhancing the compressive forces of the muscles of the abdominal cavity. Think of it this way: If you go to a baseball game and buy a well-cooked hot dog (your spine) in a very limp bun (weak abdominal muscles), the hot dog will easily flop over if pointed upward. If you gently squeeze your hand (weight-lifting belt) around the bun, this offers much better upright support.

Since overuse of weight-lifting belts can weaken the abdominals by doing their work for them, it is recommended that a belt be worn *only* when very heavy weight is to be supported above the waistline in any way, including standing, sitting, or especially bending over. In addition, belts should not be used at all for lighter lifts. Although the belt can be effective, *it is not a replacement for good technique and strong abdominal and spinal muscles.*

> "Strength training suffers from the image of overdeveloped men and women showing off their muscles. But it has real benefits for people of all ages and sizes."
> —Terrie Rizzo

be overtraining. These may also be symptoms of illness. If you are not sure, see your physician. Remember, focus on increases in strength, not soreness, to gauge your progress. If you are nott getting stronger, you are probably doing something wrong.

USE GOOD BODY MECHANICS You may not have a bad back now, but if you don't use proper body mechanics when lifting weights—even a pencil!—from the floor, you soon will. Improper body mechanics can place undue stress on the lower back and cause either immediate or latent problems in the spinal musculoskeletal system. For instructions on how to lift anything correctly, see the chapter Keeping Your Back Healthy.

Pain and Soreness

The effect of strength training can be thought of as breaking down the muscle tissue during exercise, and rebuilding it stronger during rest. As a result of the exercise, some mild soreness and discomfort is common when beginning or increasing *any* exercise routine, especially if you have been sedentary.

Although the specifics of muscular soreness are not clearly understood, soreness after exercise commonly indicates that the body is rebuilding and not ready to perform maximally. If you are sore, exercise mildly or not at all.

NO BRAIN, NO GAIN You've probably heard this one: "If it doesn't hurt the next day, you didn't exercise hard enough —no pain, no gain." Not only is this untrue, it's a dangerous philosophy. Because as muscular fitness increases, even as you lift heavier weights, you will experience less post-exercise soreness over time. Thus it is conceivable that as you become more fit, you may increase your chances of exercising far beyond your limits in order to create great muscular soreness, and this may invite injury.

Extreme soreness after exercise is not the goal of strength training; increasing strength is. If you become very sore, this means you have overdone it. Consider it a lesson learned and go easy on yourself next time. Besides, who looks forward to an exercise routine that is guaranteed to hurt? Use your head: No brain, no gain.

PAIN: BEYOND SORENESS   If severe or chronic pain occurs or persists either during or after exercise, see your physician or other qualified personnel. You may be advised to perform such measures as a proper warm-up, lift with a lighter resistance, exercise in a range of motion that does not elicit pain, or stop the particular exercise causing you pain. Complete abstinence from exercise altogether is usually not necessary. When in doubt, apply this rule of thumb: If it hurts, don't do it.

The Four Keys to Proper Form

Correctly performing strength exercises depends on four basic concepts of form. Maintaining proper form is more important than lifting more weight, because it will help you avoid injury, wasted effort, and precious time.

1. Go through a complete range of motion.
2. Move slowly and steadily.

Myth: **Weight lifting makes women look masculine.**

Fact: **Women who lift weights can increase their strength and tone without bulking up.**

3. Breathe!

4. Maintain a neutral spine.

These keys seem simple, but they can be difficult during actual exercise because their application will differ with each exercise. As you learn for the first time, or eventually begin to experiment with greater loads, be sure to maintain proper form by taking a little inventory of these four basic concepts. If you find that your form is suffering, the load is too heavy.

COMPLETE RANGE OF MOTION Unless you exercise through the entire range of motion, you will not tend to build strength in the entire muscle, but only the part of the muscle being used. To exercise the entire muscle, you have to exercise through the entire range of motion.

In each exercise, you should feel that you are developing a complete tension as the resistance is raised, progressively easing into a complete relaxation or stretch as it is lowered.

MOVE SLOWLY AND STEADILY Rocketing through a motion while grasping onto a weight creates very sharp ballistic forces that act on the joints, muscles, ligaments, and tendons of all the joints involved. This is especially true at the bottom of the range of motion where the weight must be slowed, stopped, and sped back upward against gravity in a sharp snapping action, like a bungee cord. This can invite tearing or damage of any of the associated structures.

Proper weight-training technique must employ the use of slow and steady motions. *If it feels too slow, that is the perfect speed.* It should be the speed of pulling *thick* taffy—about two seconds up and two seconds down.

BREATHE! As you fatigue during exercise, your body's capacity to produce energy will greatly diminish, at least if you are doing things right. Because the body utilizes little oxygen while lifting, proper breathing technique during the lift is important—not for the body's need for oxygen, but due to biomechanics. Thus your ability to continue the activity will depend on how efficiently you use your energy.

The most efficient use of your energy while strength training is accomplished by *separating* the most exertive phases of breathing (inhalation) and lifting (raising the weight) so that they do not compete simultaneously for your finite supply of energy. *To do this, exhale when the weight rises, "blow it away" and inhale when the weight lowers.* Here's another way to remember: Before lifting anything, inhale deeply first. This way, you have no choice but to exhale when you raise the resistance.

Exhale evenly as you raise the weight, not after you get there, as though you have sprung a leak. You want to economize your efforts so that you stop the exercise due to tiring muscles, not bad form. Otherwise, you will be working against yourself.

Always avoid holding your breath during heavy resistance exercise. Such forced breath holding is called the Valsalva maneuver. This action can temporarily raise blood pressure —sometimes so severely that the normal blood pressure of 120/80 mm Hg can rise to a dangerous level of up to 300/ 200 mm or Hg. Also, the Valsalva maneuver decreases blood flow back to the heart. If you have chronic high blood pressure or another cardiovascular condition, the Valsalva maneuver can stress your cardiovascular system well beyond a safe point and increase your chances of having a cardiovascular accident. If fact, if you have high blood pressure, you should not be performing heavy resistance training. (See the chapter Controlling High Blood Pressure with Exercise for more appropriate exercises.) When the Valsalva maneuver is preceded by rapid hyperventilation, fainting can occur. *In short, don't hold your breath.*

MAINTAIN A NEUTRAL SPINE   Neutral spine is the same as keeping your back straight; but since the spine has three natural curvatures when erect, the word straight might be misleading. In neutral spine, the spinal column is in an upright stack, like a stack of poker chips, and can be very strong and stable. Deviating from this position by bending or arching under load can cause severe forces on the spinal column and put you at risk for injury.

If you lay against a bench and relax, you will be in neutral spine. However, when standing, you have no reference point. To find neutral spine while standing, relax your neck and balance your head over your shoulders. Then relax your torso and balance your shoulders over your hips. Finally, like Elvis, rock your hips all the way forward and then backward. Find a comfortable center point, and that should do it. When bending or stooping, try to maintain this position by bending at the hips and legs, not the spine, and keeping your chest forward, your head up, and your rear end pushed back. Whenever possible, bend the knees instead of the spine.

A Few More Things to Keep in Mind

Before you begin, we'd like to leave you with a few final reminders:

- *Know your limits.* If you are not sure whether you can hold a certain amount of weight above your waistline, try less weight until you are confident that you can lift the heavier weight.

- *Avoid bending far backward (hyperextending the spine) past the point that your body is straight.* Don't lift heavy weights while bent over unless you have at least one hand down to support the weight. A special lifting belt may also be worn for safety (see "A Word About Lifting Belts").

- *Never attempt ballistic spinal twisting motions under load.* If you really want to destroy your spine in the quickest, most efficient manner, bend over with a heavy weight and twist as hard as you can! The twisting action can create tremendous shearing action that can destroy intervertebral discs in the spine. Don't twist the spine under load!

Strength-Training Exercises

Here are some general training tips for the strength exercises in this section:

1. Work slowly and with control, concentrating on the muscles you are contracting.

2. Work through a full range of motion for each exercise unless the instructions call for a shorter range.

3. Never sacrifice form to add more weight, move faster, or complete more repetitions than you are capable of doing.

4. Evaluate the amount of weight you need to use for each muscle group separately. For example, you may want to use weights for some exercises but not for others.

Note that some instructions call for use of light weights. If you don't have weights, use soup cans or other light hand-sized objects. If you prefer not to use weights, just use self-resistance!

SUPINE DUMBBELL PRESS   *Focus: Front of shoulders and arms.* Lying on your back or on a step, start with hands/ weights at shoulders. Slowly press hands/ weights up toward the ceiling from the shoulders. Lower back down slowly to the shoulders.

SUPINE DUMBBELL FLY   *Focus: Chest, front of shoulders, and arms.* Lying on your back or on a step, start with arms out to the sides and elbows slightly bent. Keeping elbows slightly bent, slowly bring weights together over the chest. Return to sides.

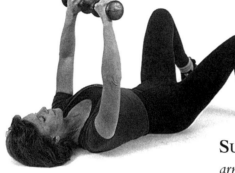

SUPINE DUMBBELL PRESS
Slowly press weights up toward the ceiling from the shoulders.

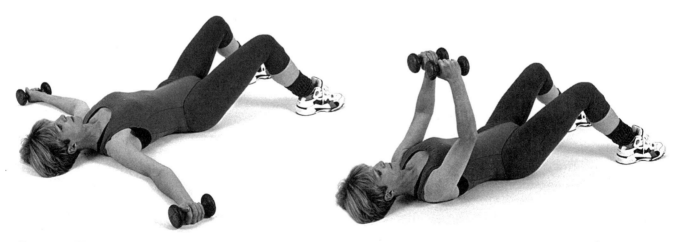

SUPINE DUMBBELL FLY
Start with arms out to the sides and elbows slightly bent.

Keeping elbows slightly bent, slowly bring hands/weights together over the chest.

Prone Back Fly *Focus: Mid-back.* Lie on your stomach on step or bench. Start with weights or hands on the floor on both sides. Lift weights/hand up to shoulder height, pulling the shoulder blades together and keeping elbows up. Return to sides.

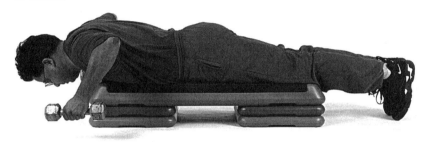

Prone Back Fly

Lift weights up to shoulder height, pulling the shoulder blades together and keeping elbows up.

Lateral Shoulder Raise
(can be done seated or standing)
Focus: Shoulders.
Start with weights/hands at the side of the body. Lift the weights/hands up laterally to a point just below shoulder height. Return to sides.

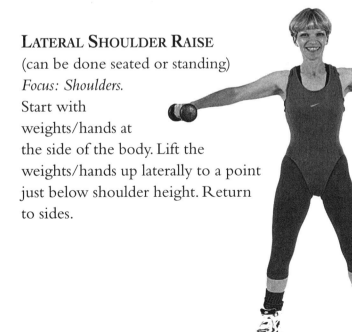

Lateral Shoulder Raise

Lift the weights/hands up laterally to a point just below shoulder height.

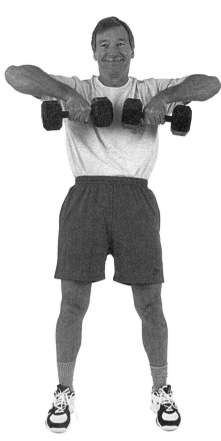

UPRIGHT ROW   *Focus: Upper back and shoulders.* Stand with weights or hands in front of hips. Lift weights/hands straight up to the chin with elbows raising to the sides.

TRICEPS PRESS   (can be done standing or using bench for support) *Focus: Triceps (back of upper arm).* Start with one hand on knee or bench for support, the other foot back on the floor for stability, and the weight/hand straight down to the floor. Raise weight/hand up to hip by bending elbow; then straighten elbow; bend elbow, while returning weight/hand to hip; straighten elbow to starting position.

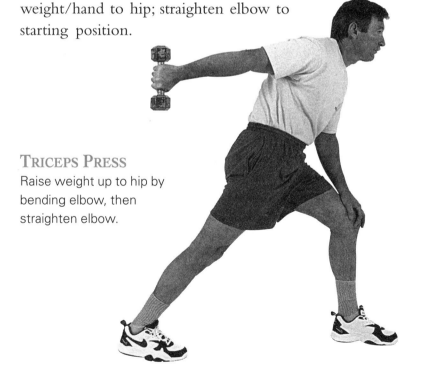

UPRIGHT ROW
Lift weights straight up to the chin with elbows raising to the sides.

TRICEPS PRESS
Raise weight up to hip by bending elbow, then straighten elbow.

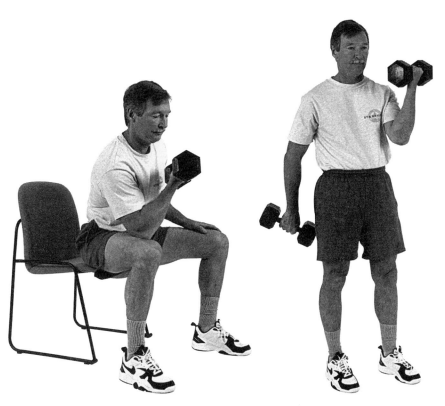

BICEPS CURLS
Bending at elbow, raise weight to the shoulder.

BICEPS CURLS (can be done standing or seated) *Focus: Biceps (front of upper arm).* Start with weights/hands by sides. Keep elbows close to body. Bending at elbow, raise one weight at a time to the shoulder; slowly lower to starting position. Alternate sides or do sets on one side at a time.

ROTATOR CUFF PRESS *Focus: Shoulder rotator cuff.* Start lying on one hip with elbow propping up the upper body, weight in other hand. Bend knees and hips to be at right angles to the body for stability. Starting with weight/hand on the ground in front of body and elbow fixed into top hip, raise the weight up above the shoulder. Lower slowly to starting position. *Note: The movement comes from the shoulder, not the elbow or back.*

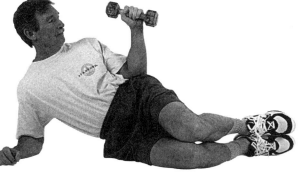

ROTATOR CUFF PRESS
Starting with weight on the ground in front of body and elbow fixed into top hip, raise the weight up above the shoulder.

MODIFIED PUSH-UPS *Focus: Upper body, particularly chest and arms.* On hands and knees, "walk" hands forward until weight is forward of (not on) kneecaps and back is straight. Keep knees close together and lightly cross ankles. Consciously contract abdominals, buttocks, and lower back to "lock" in neutral position. Bend elbows to lower upper body toward floor; straighten arms to return body to starting position. *Caution: Be careful not to arch back or extend head forward when lowering. Be careful not to hyperextend arms on return.*

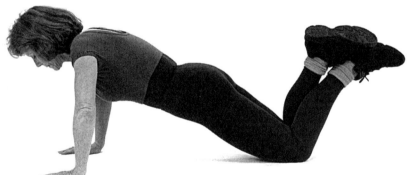

MODIFIED PUSH-UPS

Keep knees close together and lightly cross ankles. Consciously contract abdominals, buttocks, and lower back to "lock" in neutral position. Bend elbows to lower upper body; return.

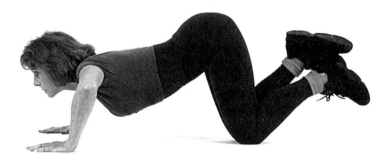

BAD PUSH-UP

Be careful not to arch back or extend head forward when lowering. Be careful not to hyperextend arms on return.

QUARTER- OR HALF-SQUAT *Focus: Lower body, particularly front and back of thighs, buttocks.* Start with legs apart and toes pointing forward. Slowly bend knees as if you were going to sit back in a chair until your thighs are semi-parallel to the floor. As you "sit," lift your arms forward to shoulder height to help maintain good alignment. Do not bend knees to more than a 90-degree angle or allow knees to extend past toes   (Knees should remain directly above or slightly in front of ankles.) Slowly return to upright. *Note: The quarter- or half-squat is an excellent exercise for strengthening the muscles of the lower body if care is taken to perform the movement correctly, and if the movement does not cause discomfort to the knees. Carefully observe the rules for correct body alignment when doing this exercise. If you feel discomfort, substitute other exercises such as Quadriceps Lifts, Hamstring Curls, and Buttocks Squeezes.*

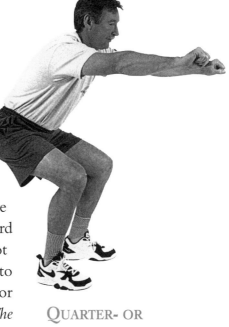

QUARTER- OR HALF-SQUAT
As you "sit," lift your arms forward to shoulder height to help maintain good alignment.

SEATED QUADRICEPS LIFT *Focus: Front of thigh; also strengthens knee.* Start seated on floor, bench, or chair. Keeping abdominal muscles contracted for stability and one leg bent, extend other leg forward. Lift extended leg several inches. Return and repeat set with other leg. *Caution: Be sure to keep back straight. Do not round back or slump forward.*

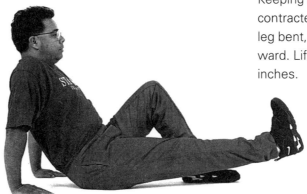

SEATED QUADRICEPS LIFT
Keeping abdominal muscles contracted for stability and one leg bent, extend other leg forward. Lift extended leg several inches.

SIDE LEG LIFTS *Focus: Outer thighs.* Start on right side with toes pointing forward, right leg slightly bent for stability, head resting on right arm. Place left hand on floor in front of chest and extend left leg straight down with foot lightly flexed. Keeping hips "stacked," lift left leg straight up to slightly above hip height (no higher than 45 degrees) and hold two seconds. Lower leg to starting position. Repeat with other leg. *Caution: Keep the hip, knee, and side of ankle aligned and facing ceiling, and do not let hips roll forward or back.*

SIDE LEG LIFTS

Keeping hips "stacked," lift left leg straight up to slightly above hip height and hold two seconds.

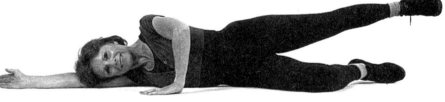

SIDE "CHAIR-POSITION" LIFT *Focus: Outer thighs and upper hips.* Start on right side in "chair" position—both knees bent and lower legs perpendicular, as if seated in a chair—with head resting on right arm. Place left hand on floor in front of chest for stability. Keeping hips "stacked," lift left leg up to slightly above hip height and hold two seconds. Lower leg, being sure not to touch knees. Repeat set with other leg. *Caution: Be careful not to lift knee past a 45-degree angle.*

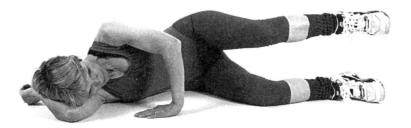

SIDE "CHAIR-POSITION" LIFT

Keeping hips "stacked," lift left leg up to slightly above hip height and hold two seconds.

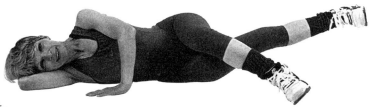

INNER THIGH LIFT *Focus: Inner thighs.* Start on right side with bottom (right) leg extended straight, head lying on right arm. Place left hand in front of chest for stability. Bring top (left) leg forward in flexed position, with weight on the inside edge of the foot, knee lifted to stay at the same plane as the left hip joint. Keeping the inside of the foot to the ceiling, lift the bottom (left) leg up several inches. Lower. Repeat set with other leg. *Caution: Be careful not to let hips roll forward or back or let toes point toward ceiling.*

INNER THIGH LIFT
Keeping the inside of the foot to the ceiling, lift the bottom leg up several inches.

DECLINE HAMSTRING BRIDGE *Focus: Hamstrings and buttocks.* Start on back with hands to sides, right heel on the left knee, and left foot on floor with knee bent. Maintaining a neutral spine, press through right heel to lift your hips slightly off floor. Contract buttocks at the top of the lift. Lower to starting position.

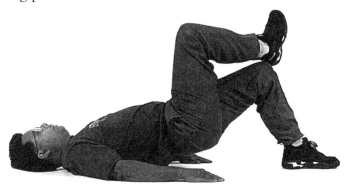

DECLINE HAMSTRING BRIDGE
Maintaining a neutral spine, press through heel to lift your hips slightly off floor.

BUTTOCKS CONTRACTIONS *Focus: Buttocks.* Start on back with both knees bent and hands on abdomen. Contract abs to tilt pelvis forward to "tuck" position. Lift hips one or two inches off floor. Contract buttocks muscles and hold two seconds. Release contraction without lowering hips. *Note: Be careful not to lift buttocks too high or overarch back.*

BUTTOCKS CONTRACTIONS
Lift hips one or two inches off floor. Contract buttocks muscles and hold two seconds.

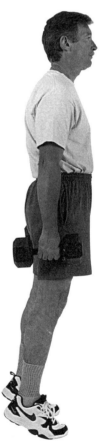

STANDING CALF RAISE *Focus: Calves.* Start with both feet on the floor, hip-width apart. Slowly rise to balls of feet. Hold. Slowly lower heels slightly, but not to floor. Repeat five times before lowering heels to floor. Do several sets of five lifts. *Note: Be careful to keep knees "soft" and ankles straight—don't roll your ankles or shift weight to the outside of your feet. This exercise is especially beneficial for older adults, to help maintain strength in the calf muscles.*

STANDING CALF RAISE
Slowly rise to balls of feet. Hold.

STANDING DIP *Focus: Quadriceps, hamstrings, buttocks, and calves.* Starting with feet together, take a giant step backward and slightly to the side with right foot, keeping heel up. Keep left foot flat on the floor, knee in line over ankle and spine in neutral position. Place hands on front of right thigh for support. Lean slightly forward to shift weight over your front (left) thigh. Maintaining torso position and keeping hips square, lower or "dip" left knee several inches to floor. Return. Repeat with other side. *Note: As with squats, be careful to maintain correct knee and body alignment; substitute other exercises if you notice knee discomfort.*

REAR LIFT *Focus: Buttocks and hamstrings.* Start on all fours (elbows and knees), with elbows directly below shoulders and knees directly below hips. Keep head/neck in neutral position and abdominals tight for stability. Extend left leg directly back, resting on floor. Keeping abdominals tight, contract buttocks to lift heel to buttocks height. Lower foot to floor. Do repetitions, then repeat with other leg. *Note: Be sure not to raise one hip higher than the other hip.*

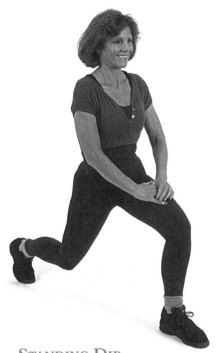

STANDING DIP
Maintaining torso position and keeping hips square, lower or "dip" knee several inches to floor.

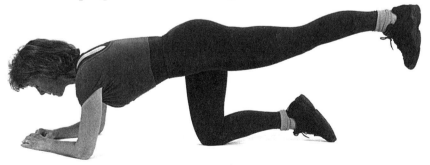

REAR LIFT
Keeping abdominals tight, contract buttocks to lift heel to buttocks height.

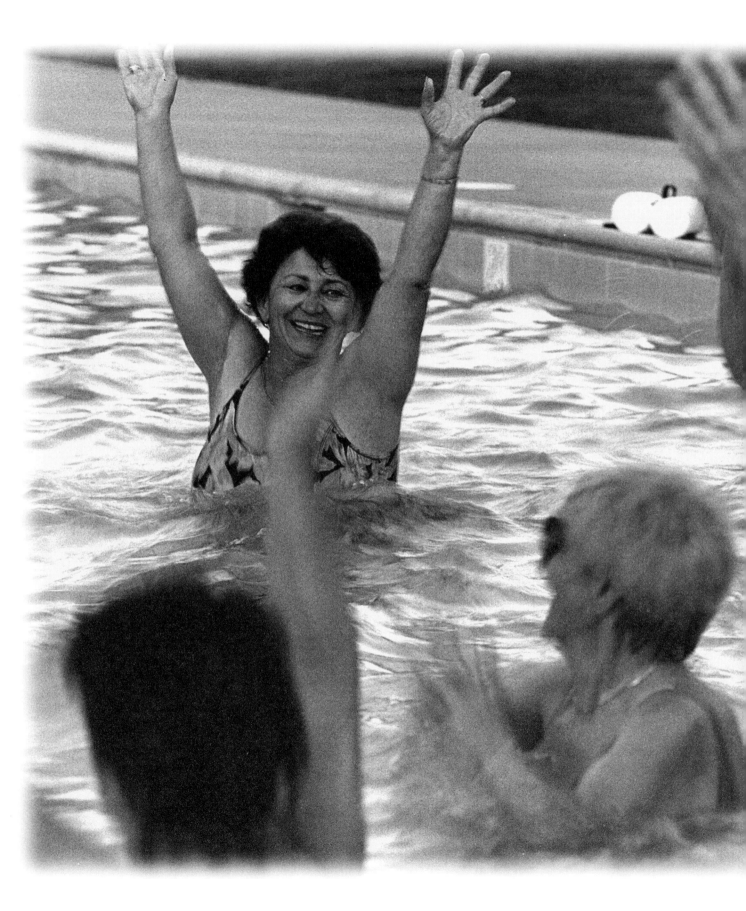

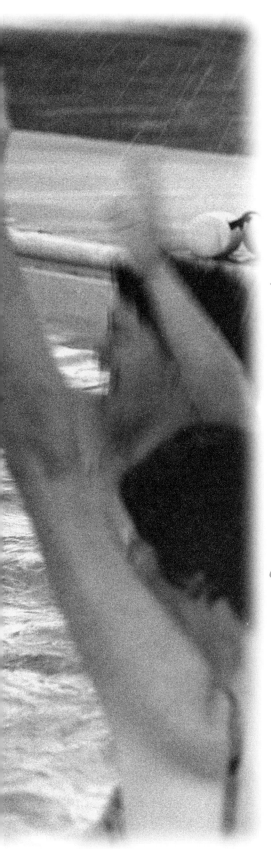

Part Three

*E*xercise for Special Needs

"No matter what your physical problems, you can benefit from regular exercise. You can adapt most activities to suit your needs. You may have to begin more slowly, with fewer exercises, or with changes in equipment—but the important thing is to get started and keep it up."

—Terrie Rizzo

Exercising After a *Heart* Attack

Robert F. DeBusk, M.D.
C. Barr Taylor, M.D.

By three weeks after a heart attack, most patients can return to their previous level of exercise. After six to twelve weeks of exercise training, many actually perform better than they could before their heart attack.

*I*N THE PAST, PEOPLE WHO HAD suffered a heart attack (that is, a myocardial infarction, or M.I.) were confined to bed for six weeks and were frequently unable to resume exercise until at least three months after the event. However, significant advances in medical research have brought a much fuller understanding of the processes involved in recovery.

Today we know that by three weeks after an attack, the heart has already healed sufficiently to sustain considerable exercise. By this time, most patients can be assured by their doctors that they can resume their normal lives and return to their previous level of exercise without worry.

Approximately 600,000 people survive heart attacks each year. Of these, about 75 percent can undergo formal exercise training based on the fact they are at low risk for another heart attack, have undergone balloon angioplasty or coronary bypass surgery to reduce risk, and have no limiting medical or musculoskeletal conditions.

Exercise Helps Recovery

The benefits of exercise for a person who has had a heart attack are similar to the exercise benefits most healthy people enjoy. Exercise helps reduce weight, blood pressure, and stress. Moreover, exercise may increase the beneficial type of cholesterol, HDL, especially in those who exercise regularly.

Regular exercise also has benefits that are of special significance to people who have had heart attacks—psychological improvement and the reduced demand for oxygen by the heart as it becomes more efficient. Not surprisingly, after a

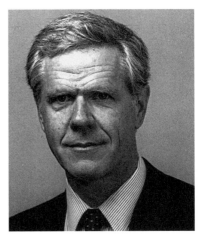

Robert F. DeBusk, M.D., is Professor of Medicine, Stanford Medical School, and Director, Stanford Cardiac Rehabilitation Program. For exercise, he enjoys road cycling.

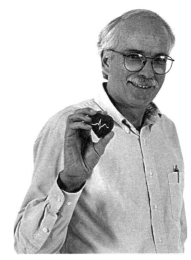

C. Barr Taylor, M.D., is Professor of Psychiatry at Stanford Medical School, Co-Director of the Stanford Cardiac Rehabilitation Program, and Director of Behavioral Science for the Stanford Heart Disease Prevention Program. He is an avid fly fisherman, and enjoys walking, playing basketball, and skiing.

Are You Ready for Exercise?

The treadmill test—which measures the heart's capacity to tolerate a wide variety of stresses of daily life—is an invaluable tool. As early as five days after a heart attack, doctors can determine patients' risk for future heart attack or death, based on their medical history and clinical tests.

If the results of a treadmill test given two to three weeks after the heart attack show an absence of oxygen deprivation to the heart and good pumping function, the patient can generally be classified as low risk. *This includes at least half of all post-M.I. patients.* For patients in the low-risk category, the risk of dying from a heart attack is less than 2 percent a year. That increased confidence can itself be a major factor in ensuring recovery.

Low-risk patients can be immediately cleared for exercise training, which will in itself increase their confidence to engage in other activities, such as rapid walking, yard work, and sexual relations. Just getting back to these normal daily activities brings about additional physical and psychological benefits.

If you are recovering from a heart attack, a treadmill test can help define your medical prognosis and give you realistic expectations about your ability to resume your customary activities.

heart attack many people are anxious and uncertain about their ability to resume work and other activities. They may be depressed if they are unduly restricted from these activities. As they become more physically active through exercise, and see their own capabilities return, depression tends to dissipate and their anxiety is relieved.

Exercise also causes physiological changes that can enhance the feeling of well-being. As the heart rate decreases from exercise training, the heart muscle becomes more efficient. Patients suffering symptoms of angina (lack of oxygen to the heart muscle) often find that their symptoms diminish or disappear altogether. As a result, they find that they are able to carry out physical activities without discomfort.

Getting Back to Exercise

Within three months of a heart attack, the low-risk patient has an exercise capacity that is equivalent to that of a healthy person between the ages of fifty and fifty-nine. These men and women can safely embark on an exercise program similar to that recommended for any beginner. Today, most doctors recommend twenty to thirty minutes a day of walking, cycling, and jogging at 60 percent to 75 percent of the peak heart rate.

HOME-BASED EXERCISE   In the past, post-M.I. patients typically exercised in a group setting under medical supervision. However, the treadmill test has enabled us to reevaluate that approach.

In a random trial of clinically low-risk patients, the Stanford Cardiac Rehabilitation Program assigned half to exercise at home, and half to exercise in a supervised group. Both groups were given individualized guidelines for exercise intensity based on a treadmill evaluation at three weeks after the heart attack. Patients training at home used heart-rate monitors to help them stay within the prescribed range of intensity. Program nurses phoned them periodically to discuss their adherence to exercise and any problems they encountered. A total of 78 percent of patients participated in home-based training, 63 percent starting at three weeks, and 15 percent after undergoing coronary bypass surgery or balloon angioplasty—on average, eight to twelve weeks after a heart attack.

The results were encouraging for anyone who is considering resuming exercise after a heart attack: No training-related cardiac events were noted. Home-based exercise training proved just as effective—and just as safe—as supervised group training.

Myth: It's not safe to exercise —people are always having heart attacks while running.

Fact: People have heart attacks because of underlying coronary artery disease, not because of exercise. Moreover, at least one-third of patients who die suddenly during exercise have prior clinical evidence of coronary artery disease.

Safety First!

As with any exercise program, safety is primary. Resist the tendency to overwork, and don't ignore any unusual symptoms.

It's important to be in touch with your body's feelings. Use your self-monitoring skills to be alert for any warning signals:

> **"Exercise is an important part of your recovery process. Make sure you have medical approval, and don't be afraid to renew your physical activity."** —Terrie Rizzo

- chest discomfort
- undue fatigue
- shortness of breath
- irregular pulse or heartbeat

If you feel any of these, stop exercising and contact your doctor. Your ability to recognize a change in symptoms and to seek medical attention is critical to ensuring the safety of continued exercise.

If you are a post-M.I. patient exercising at home, observe these common-sense precautions:

- Regulate the intensity of your exercise within your own limits.
- Stop exercising if you do not feel well.
- Monitor your heart rate while exercising by checking your pulse to make sure it is within the range suggested by your doctor.

In our program, we do our best to ensure safety by selecting only appropriate patients and helping them to develop self-monitoring skills. To a great extent, safety is in the hands of each patient. When you exercise with common sense and self-awareness, your program will enhance your recovery and add to a full and healthy life.

Controlling *High Blood Pressure* with Exercise

Stephen P. Fortmann, M.D.

More and more doctors today are suggesting lifestyle changes—including exercise—before they prescribe drugs to lower blood pressure.

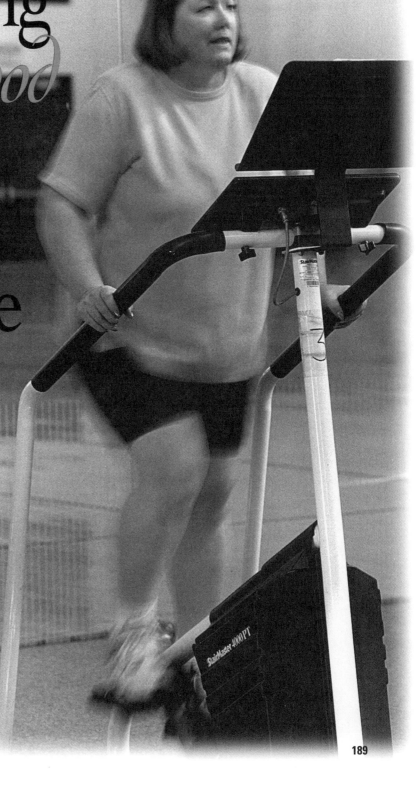

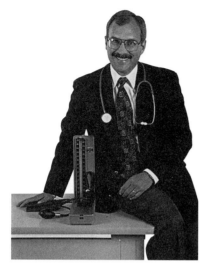

Stephen P. Fortmann, M.D., is Deputy Director, Stanford Center for Research in Disease Prevention; Associate Professor, Department of Medicine, Stanford Medical School; and Director of the Stanford Preventive Cardiology Clinic. For exercise, he says, "I run. My eleven-year-old English Brittany accompanies me, exploring thoroughly the scents we pass such that she and I conduct a daily game of the tortoise and the hare (I needn't mention which of us is the tortoise)."

A FEW YEARS AGO, if you were diagnosed with hypertension—chronic high blood pressure—your doctor would probably have sent you home with a prescription for medication and the advice to take it easy. Increasingly, I am glad to say, physicians suggest changes in lifestyle before they resort to drugs. These measures often include:

- a reduction in weight
- a reduction in salt, which can have a distinct effect on those susceptible to it
- a reduction in alcohol, which can raise pressure in certain people
- a less stressful existence
- exercise

Why exercise? Because even though we don't know precisely how exercise has an independent effect on blood pressure levels, it can definitely help reduce them. In many cases, the main benefit of exercise will come from its effect on weight, or perhaps on stress. And there is now some evidence that exercise alone does indeed have some independent effect on pressure.

How High Is High?

What we call "high" blood pressure is now somewhat lower than it used to be. Thanks to long-term studies, blood pressure that was considered "within normal limits" ten years ago is now considered risky. Quite simply, we have found that even mild elevation of pressure increases the risk of heart disease and stroke.

Blood pressure is measured in two numbers, *systolic* (the high number recorded when your heart is actually beating) and *diastolic* (the low number, indicating the pressure between beats). The change in attitude toward the systolic pressure has been particularly dramatic. Not long ago, a systolic pressure of your age plus 100 was considered respectable. Today that formula is considered too high over the age of twenty! In fact, we now think that the systolic should stay at or below 120 for life, and that anything over 140 should be carefully evaluated by a physician.

Meanwhile, diastolic pressure should ideally stay at 80 or below for life. Most physicians now express concern with any diastolic pressure above 90 or 95.

So, while there is much variation from moment to moment, the ideal average blood pressure is 120/80 or below. Most doctors tend to prescribe drugs for people whose pressure is consistently higher than 150/100, especially if the person has elevated cholesterol levels or smokes cigarettes. People who stick to the proper exercise program, however, can see dramatic improvement in blood pressure.

How Exercise Affects Blood Pressure

The connection between exercise and blood pressure is complex. Indeed, blood pressure is affected by so many factors that good research studies must have a control group to ensure that changes in blood pressure can be attributed solely to exercise rather than to factors such as weight loss.

One study that did make good use of a control group was performed by Dr. Steven Blair and his colleagues at the Institute for Aerobics Research in Dallas. They studied fifty-six young people with mild hypertension, of whom twelve acted as controls and went about their lives with no change. The other forty-four participated in a program of three sixty-minute walk/jog sessions a week for a period of sixteen weeks.

The results were very interesting for the exercisers. Although their weight did not change, their average blood pressure declined from 146/94 to 134/87. In the control group, whose weight also remained stable, the systolic pressure also dropped from an average of 145 to 138, but the group's diastolic pressure did not decline during the sixteen-week trial (indeed, it went up by an average of three points). Clearly, the exercise program appeared to have a more significant effect on the diastolic than on the systolic pressure.

Several other controlled studies do exist, and the best guess at this time is that exercise does have a modest, independent blood-pressure-lowering effect. Added to its positive effect on weight and stress, the total benefit of exercise on blood pressure control becomes considerably greater.

How Weight Affects Blood Pressure

Excess weight plays an important role in blood pressure. In fact, for many people, it is more beneficial to lose weight than to cut down on sodium (although in an ideal world, they do both).

While most people who reduce their salt intake will lower their blood pressure, some will not. But almost all people with

> *"A few years ago, doctors didn't recommend exercise for hypertensive patients, but we know now that regular exercise is a key element of blood pressure control. "*—**Terrie Rizzo**

chronic high blood pressure will reduce their pressure if they lose weight—usually at the rate of about one point of systolic pressure for each one or two pounds lost. And exercise is a vital component in almost all successful weight-loss programs.

THE EXERCISE CONNECTION   Clearly, exercise uses up calories and therefore allows you to eat a reasonable amount of food while losing weight. But it also influences two other important factors in weight loss: the type of weight that you lose (whether fat or muscle), and your basic resting metabolism.

Any weight-loss program that relies for its effectiveness on a reduction in calories alone will remove surplus flab from your frame, but it will also diminish your stock of lean muscle tissue. Since muscle tissue uses up more calories than flab, its loss will make it harder for you to keep the weight off when you go back to your normal way of eating.

On the other hand, if part or all of your weight loss comes from an increase in exercise, you will be building more muscle tissue, and that will increase your body's capacity to use up incoming calories without going on a starvation diet. Some exciting research in the last decade has indicated that a systematic program of aerobic exercise can speed up the basic metabolic rate, or BMR. Thanks to a hopped-up BMR, the "trained" person will use up more calories than the untrained, even while resting.

Related to this, perhaps, is the discovery that the "appetite alarms" in the exercised person are more reliable than in the nonexerciser. A program of systematic exercise may increase the likelihood that when you feel hungry, you are hungry; and that will make it somewhat easier to resist the high-fat snacks that are the nemesis of most dieters. There is evidence that moderate exercise, such as a brisk walk before dinner, can actually reduce the appetite. For more information, see the chapter Eat Well, Be Well.

How Stress Affects Blood Pressure

Stress certainly can be a factor in chronic hypertension, and it definitely can boost blood pressure temporarily. The shot of adrenalin that comes with any sudden excitement, preparing us for "fight or flight," speeds up the heart rate and increases blood pressure. In people with normal blood pressure, the pressure goes back down again as soon as the emergency is over. But some investigators believe that chronic stress helps create changes in the body that produce sustained blood pressure elevation.

Several studies have shown small reductions in blood pressure with regular stress-reduction efforts. A program that reduces stress, be it meditation, yoga, or exercise, may make a useful addition to a program for the control of high blood pressure. For more information, see the chapter Mind + Body: The No-Stress Equation.

THE EXERCISE CONNECTION   How does exercise reduce stress? Partly through some very fancy biochemical activity in the brain. Systematic exercise can apparently increase the supply of endorphins in the bloodstream, which in turn can act as natural tranquilizers (and produce the "runner's high" that has so often been described). Endorphins can also account for the apparent reduction in stress levels that many of us experience when we are exercising.

Even without a biochemical explanation, however, there are ample reasons why exercise has a beneficial effect on stress levels. When you exercise, you are away from everyday pressures, able to let your mind roam free; you feel more in control of your body and destiny. If you exercise outdoors, you are able to appreciate some of the natural beauty around you. If you exercise with a friend or a spouse, you have a perfect setting for low-key conversation and companionship. All of this helps to control or counteract stress.

Exercising Away Your Need for Smoking, Caffeine, and Alcohol

An exercise program can bring other, less direct benefits to blood-pressure control, such as providing a substitute for smoking, caffeine, and alcohol, which all have an effect on blood pressure.

SMOKING   While quitting smoking may not reduce blood pressure, it can remove some of the danger of elevated levels. If you are trying to quit smoking, exercise can give you instant feedback on the physical improvements that come with quitting. At the very least, you'll probably notice improvements in your wind and endurance. As a bonus, you'll have a positive activity to replace the old addiction.

CAFFEINE   Caffeine may have been unjustifiably blamed where blood pressure is concerned. We know that in people who are not used to caffeine, the amount found in two cups of coffee can definitely raise blood pressure for two to three

Blood Pressure Points

Given the following precautions, a program of exercise could be the key to a long and healthy life. Use your common sense, and check with your doctor first.

1. **There are no reliable symptoms to tell you whether or not your pressure is too high.** If you don't know your pressure, have it checked before you start any vigorous exercise program. Don't rely on drugstore machines—they're not always accurate. Have it done by a health professional, preferably more than once.

2. **Don't accept a verdict of "normal for your age" or "within the normal range."** Ask for numbers, remembering that the ideal is 120/80 or less (the lower, the better). Anything over 140/90 should be taken seriously.

3. **If your blood pressure is elevated, and the doctor prescribes drugs, take them religiously.** Even if you are also taking other measures to reduce the pressure (for example, losing weight, cutting down on salt), don't stop taking the medication without being reevaluated by your physician.

4. **If your blood pressure is elevated, be particularly cautious about starting an exercise program.** It's wise to stick with walking until your pressure has come down, and your stamina has gone up enough to let you go faster without pushing your heart rate too high.

hours. We also know that since the body adjusts to caffeine, the effect disappears in regular caffeine users. So there is no compelling evidence that regular coffee or cola users need to stop if their blood pressure is high. However, some people may develop an increased sensitivity to caffeine, and it is certainly worth cutting it out for a time to see if your pressure comes down.

To be kind to yourself, stop your intake of caffeine over the course of a few days. If you cut out caffeine all at once, expect a few temporary withdrawal symptoms, such as headaches and a feeling of mental slowness. The body adjusts to the mental stimulation of caffeine, and regular users depend on it for normal mental function—which is one good reason to quit.

ALCOHOL The case against alcohol is somewhat more clear-cut. It has definitely been associated with elevated blood pressure, especially in people over age forty-five. The effect is fairly subtle, with two drinks per day increasing pressure by a few points. Clinically, we have seen people who drink more than that show marked improvement in blood pressure when they went on the wagon.

If your pressure is too high for comfort and you drink, on average, more than one cocktail, glass of wine, or bottle of beer a day, it would be wise to try reducing or stopping your drinking for three to four weeks. Then, with your doctor, assess the affect on your blood pressure. Take a walk to unwind!

Should Everyone with High Blood Pressure Exercise?

While exercise can help control many of the factors associated with high blood pressure, including weight and stress, not all people with high blood pressure should be given a blanket recommendation to exercise.

Most middle-aged Americans, for example, have some degree of blockage of their arteries. It's not a good idea to impose sudden demands for extra work on the circulatory system, particularly if there is an added risk from elevated blood pressure. You may be able to build up to a high level of activity over time; but it is important for everyone (especially those over age thirty-five) to start an exercise program slowly, and build up capacity gradually without straining the system.

What Activities Are Best?

When it comes to high blood pressure, not all exercise is equal. Certain types of exercise can actually raise blood pressure. In a healthy person, this is not necessarily harmful, since pressure will quickly return to normal. However, if pressure is already high, or even borderline, the additional load could prove dangerous.

Weight-lifting and other muscle-building exercises don't do much for blood pressure and may even raise it, at least during the effort. Maintaining muscle strength can be important, especially in the elderly, but "pumping iron" isn't going to make you much healthier.

What about aerobic exercise—-the dancing, running, brisk walking, bicycling, and swimming that raise the heartbeat and temporarily increase the workload on the whole cardiovascular system?

Not so long ago, the average cautious physician would have advised everyone with elevated blood pressure (or indeed with any hint of cardiovascular difficulty) to avoid unnecessary activity of any type. Now, however, the sight of recovered heart-attack patients and even people with heart transplants pounding along at full speed, the picture of health, has helped all but the most conservative physicians to modify their stand. Most will now permit at least a program of brisk walking. Many will encourage their patients to undertake a more vigorous exercise program, provided certain guidelines are followed:

- If you are currently being treated for high blood pressure, or have a history of high blood pressure, check with your physician before undertaking any exercise more vigorous than walking.

- Monitor your heart rate periodically during exercise (including walking).

- Always stop and rest if you feel out of breath, or if your feel any dizziness or chest pain.

- Take the talk test: Never let yourself get so out of breath that you can't hold a conversation without strain.

If you use your common sense and pay attention to the signals your body gives you, a regular program of exercise could be your key to a long and enjoyable life.

Customizing
Exercise
for
Special Needs

Kate Lorig, R.N., DR. P.H.

*Even short periods
of gentle physical
activity can signifi-
cantly improve your
health and fitness,
reduce stiffness, and
make you feel better.*

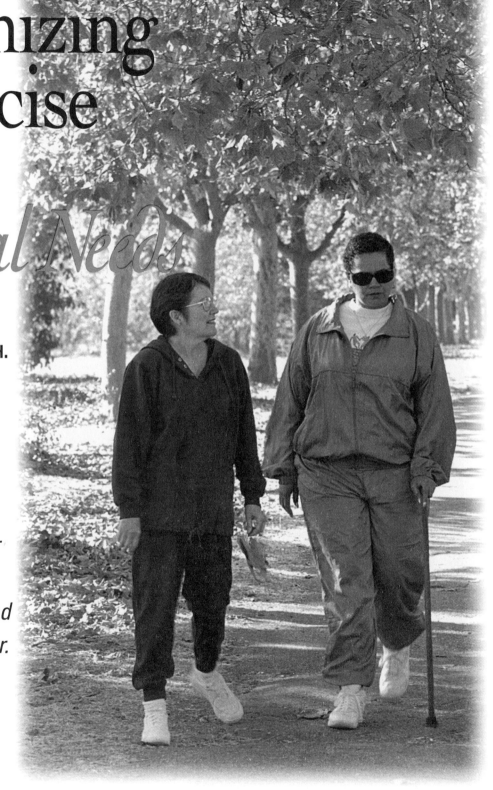

*I*F YOU HAVE RESISTED regular exercise because of chronic health problems, here's some very good news: Based on knowledge gained from many people with chronic illnesses who have participated in exercise research, we now know that regular exercise and physical activity are especially valuable to people with chronic illness—both for physical and emotional health.

Even for people in good health, long periods of inactivity can lead to weakness, fatigue, stiffness, loss of range of motion, poor appetite, constipation, obesity, depression, anxiety, and increased sensitivity to pain. For people who are dealing with chronic illness, keeping active is crucial:

- Exercising *increases* your levels of both energy and strength, and *reduces* anxiety and depression.

- Regular exercise can help you maintain a good weight, which takes stress off weight-bearing joints and improves blood pressure and blood fat levels.

- There is evidence that regular exercise can help to prevent blood clots (one of the reasons why exercise can be of particular benefit to people with heart disease, cerebrovascular disease, and peripheral vascular disease).

- For people with arthritis (and everyone else), regular exercise can help build strong muscles, which help to protect the joints by improving stability and absorbing shock. Regular exercise helps nourish joints and keep cartilage and bone healthy.

- For people with diabetes, regular exercise is an important part of controlling blood sugar levels, losing

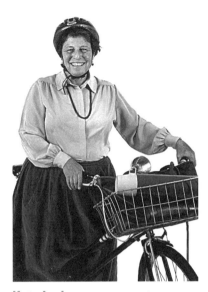

Kate Lorig, R.N., DR. P.H., is Associate Professor of Medicine (Research) at the Stanford Medical School, Director of Health Education at the Stanford Arthritis Center, and Director of Patient Education at the Stanford Patient Education Research Center. She is a committed walker and hiker for daily exercise, and she always looks for ways to include walking as part of any business trip or vacation.

"Regular exercise can help people with chronic illnesses have less pain and become more active. Go slowly, make modifications—but nearly everyone can exercise!"

—Terrie Rizzo

weight, and reducing the risks of cardiovascular complications.

- For people with chronic lung conditions, regular exercise has been shown to improve endurance and reduce shortness of breath (reducing trips to the emergency room!).

- And for many people with claudication (leg pain from severe atherosclerotic blockages in the arteries of the lower extremities), a regular exercise program improves the ability to walk farther without leg pain.

The good news is that it doesn't take hours and hours in the gym to achieve most of these health benefits. Even short periods of gentle physical activity can significantly improve health and fitness, reduce disease risks, and make you feel better. You'll be reconditioning your body, helping to restore function previously lost to disuse and illness. And this will help you improve your health and manage your chronic illness better.

The information in this and previous chapters will help you learn how to make exercise choices. However, this advice is not intended to take the place of therapeutic recommendations from your health-care provider. If an exercise plan has been prescribed for you that differs from suggestions here, take this book to your doctor or therapist and discuss everything thoroughly.

Developing Your Exercise Program

You may be surprised to learn that the basic information on exercise for people with chronic illnesses is no different than for the general population. A complete, balanced exercise program should include strength, flexibility, and aerobics. To learn more, refer to the chapters on Creating Your Own Exercise Program; Stretching for Flexibility; Get Moving, Keep Moving—Aerobically; and Using Your Muscles for Life.

FLEXIBILITY   Flexibility is the ability of the joints to move comfortably through a full, normal range of motion. It tends to diminish with inactivity, age, and certain illnesses, and limited flexibility can cause pain, increase the risk of injury, and make muscles less efficient. Most people with chronic illnesses can increase or maximize flexibility by doing gentle stretching exercises.

STRENGTH   Muscles need to be exercised to maintain strength. With inactivity, muscles tend to weaken and shrink (atrophy). Much of the disability and lack of mobility for people with chronic illness is due to muscle weakness. This can be reversed with a program of gradually increasing exercise.

AEROBIC ACTIVITY   The heart and lungs must work efficiently to distribute oxygen-rich blood to the muscles, and the muscles must be conditioned to use the oxygen. Aerobic exercise improves this cardiovascular and muscle conditioning by using the large muscles of your body in a rhythmical, continuous activity. Aerobic exercise improves cardiovascular fitness, lessens heart attack risk, and helps control weight. It also promotes a sense of "feeling good," which eases depression and anxiety, promotes restful sleep, and improves your mood and energy levels.

Preparing to Exercise

If you have a chronic illness, you may have special challenges. You must take necessary precautions and find a safe and comfortable program. However, even with chronic illness, most people can do some kind of aerobic exercise and certainly can do flexibility and strengthening exercises.

If your illness is not fairly stable, if you have been inactive for more than six months, or if you have questions about starting an aerobic exercise program, it is best to check with your doctor or therapist first. Learning how far you can push yourself without overdoing it is especially important.

Respect your body. If you feel acutely ill, don't exercise. If you can't comfortably complete your warm-up period of flexibility and strengthening exercises, then don't try to do more vigorous conditioning exercises. Your personal exercise program should be based on *your* current level of health and fitness, *your* goals and desires, *your* abilities and special needs, and *your* likes and dislikes.

Putting Your Program Together

The best way to enjoy and stick with your exercise program is to find something you like to do. Choose what you want to do, a place where you feel comfortable, and an exercise time that fits your schedule.

Pick two or three activities you think you would enjoy and that wouldn't put undue stress on your body. If an activity is new to you, try it out before going to the expense of buying equipment or joining a health club. Having several activities that you enjoy doing helps prevent boredom, and means that you can keep active while adapting to vacations, seasons, and changing problems with your illness.

Some well-meaning health professionals can make it hard for a person with chronic illness to stick to an exercise program. You may have been told simply to "exercise more on your own"—but the "how" and "when" may have been left entirely up to you. No wonder so many people never start or give up so quickly! Here are some ideas that can give you a good start on a successful program:

1. *Choose the activities that you want to do.* Combine activities your doctor or therapist recommends, some exercises from the activity chapters of this book (with approval from your own doctor), and some of your favorite activities. You don't have to do the same thing every day—in fact, that tends to be boring and reduces adherence to a program. Vary your routines to make it more interesting.

2. *Choose the time and place that you will exercise.* Choose a time and place that will work for you. Write it down, and tell your family and friends your plan. That way, you'll be more likely to stick to it. (For a sample exercise planner, see the chapter Creating Your Own Exercise Plan.)

3. *Make a contract with yourself.* Decide how long you want to stick to this specific plan—eight to twelve weeks is a reasonable time commitment for a new program. Then write down an agreement with yourself to commit that amount of time. (For an example, see the Contract for Change in the chapter No Excuses!)

4. *Write down your exercise program.* Choose your exer-

cises and write them down in a notebook so that you remember to do them each time. Make a diary or calendar and check each day that you exercise.

5. *Do some self-tests to keep track of your progress.* You will find a variety of self-tests in this book (see the table of contents for location of specific tests). Take some self-tests before you begin, and record the date and results. Continue to retake the tests periodically—you'll be amazed at your progress.

6. *Start your program.* Remember to begin gradually and proceed slowly, especially if you haven't exercised in a while.

7. *Revise your program.* At the end of your eight to twelve weeks, decide what you liked, what worked, and what made exercising difficult. Modify your program and contract for another few weeks—you may decide to change some exercises, the place or time you exercise, or your exercise partners.

8. *Expect setbacks.* During the first year, people average two to three interruptions in their exercise plans or schedules, often because of minor illnesses or injuries unrelated to their exercise. Don't be discouraged. When you are feeling better, resume your program but begin a lower, more gentle level. As a rule of thumb, it will take you the same amount of time to get back into shape as you were out. For example, if you missed two weeks, it may take at least that long to get back to your previous level. Go slowly. You are in this for the long haul.

CHOOSING A FITNESS PROGRAM   Most people who exercise regularly do so with at least one other person. On the other hand, exercising alone gives you more freedom. Either way, there are many opportunities available for exercise.

Choosing a Community Program

Look for these qualities when you choose a community fitness class or program:

1. **Classes designed for beginners that involve low- to moderate-intensity exercise.** You should be able to observe classes and participate in at least one class before paying.

2. **Certified, knowledgeable instructors.** Instructors who have knowledge and experience of a variety of problems are more likely to understand special needs and know how to make modifications you may need.

3. **Good facilities.** Choose a class that is easy to get to, park near, and enter. Dressing and exercise rooms should be accessible and safe, with professional staff on site.

For example, the Arthritis Foundation sponsors exercise programs developed specifically for people with arthritis and taught by trained instructors. The American Heart Association and the American Lung Association are excellent resources for people who have had heart disease, a stroke, or lung disease. Consult your local chapter of the appropriate agency.

Hospitals commonly offer medically supervised exercise classes for people with heart or lung disease (cardiac or pulmonary rehabilitation classes). These programs tend to be more expensive than other community classes, but they have the advantage of medical supervision, if that is important to you.

Working Out with Awareness

Exercise can work wonders, but only if you do it properly and with awareness. As you go through your program, keep in mind the suggestions in this section.

EXERCISES FOR STRENGTHENING OR FLEXIBILITY   Read the chapters on Using Your Muscles for Life and Stretching for Flexibility to learn about these exercises before you begin. As you do your stretching and strengthening exercises, always remember these points:

1. Move slowly and gently. Do not bounce or jerk.

2. Don't push your body until it hurts. Stretching should feel good, not painful.

3. Start slowly, generally with no more than five repetitions of any exercise. Take at least two weeks to increase to ten repetitions.

4. Arrange your exercises so you don't have to get up or down off the floor often.

5. Always do the same number of exercises for your left side as for your right side.

6. Muscle or joint pain that lasts more than two hours after the exercise, or feeling tired into the next day, means that you probably did too much too fast. *Don't quit exercising!* Next time just do fewer repetitions, or eliminate an exercise that seems to be causing the symptoms.

7. Any exercise can be adapted to your individual needs. If you are limited by muscle weakness or joint tightness, remember that you don't have to complete a movement perfectly. The benefit of an exercise comes from doing it to the best of your ability.

AEROBIC ACTIVITIES   The chapter Get Moving, Keep Moving—Aerobically will tell you all about aerobics. The activity you choose will depend on your needs, limitations, and preferences. The following, however, are particularly good for people with a variety of health problems.

Walking. Walking is a good aerobic choice for many people with a chronic illness. Using a cane or walker need not stop you from getting into a walking routine. (If you are in a wheelchair, use crutches, or experience more than mild discomfort when you walk a short distance, you should consider some other type of aerobic exercise, or consult a physician or therapist for help.)

If you haven't been doing much for a while, ten minutes of walking may be enough. Build up your time by no more than five minutes each week until you are up to twenty or thirty minutes. Follow the frequency, duration, and intensity guidelines outlined in the aerobics chapter.

Water exercise. Swimming and water aerobics are other good forms of endurance exercise, and may put less stress on joints. For most people with chronic illness, these are excellent choices since they use the whole body. You even can sit in a chair in fairly shallow water to do water exercise.

For people with asthma, swimming can be a preferred form of exercise because the moisture helps reduce shortness of breath. However, since swimming involves the arms, it can lead to excessive shortness of breath in people with lung disease.

People with heart disease who have severely irregular heartbeats and have had an implantable "defibrillator" (AIDC) permanently implanted in their hearts should avoid swimming.

If you have had a stroke, or have another condition that may affect your strength and balance, make sure that you have someone to help you in and out of the pool. Find a position close to the wall or a "buddy" to add to your safety and security.

Stationary cycling. Stationary bicycling is another good form of aerobic exercise for people with chronic illnesses. It doesn't excessively strain the hips, knees, and feet if done correctly, and you can easily adjust how hard you work.

Low-impact aerobic dance. If you do low-impact aerobics, you can make modifications based on your needs. You can pace yourself by slowing down or walking in place.

Exercise Tips for Specific Chronic Illnesses

Here are a few specific recommendations for people with specific health problems. Always consult your health practitioner to discuss your own special needs.

LUNG DISEASE Exercise training has been found to increase endurance, improve symptoms, and reduce hospital visits for people with chronic lung disease. Your exercise routine should begin at a *very* low intensity, with a very gradual increase in your activity. With time, you'll notice that the shortness of breath at a given level of exercise will start to decrease. Work with your doctor to plan the safest, most beneficial exercise program for you.

Use your medicine, particularly your inhaler, *before you exercise.* It will help you exercise longer and with less shortness of breath.

If you become severely short of breath with only minimal exertion, your doctor may want to change your medicine, or even have you use supplemental oxygen before you begin your conditioning exercises.

Be sure to warm up and cool down gradually, taking adequate time, when doing conditioning activities. Remember

Self-Test: Dyspnea Index

Dyspnea refers to shortness of breath. The dyspnea index measures exercise intensity according to the amount of respiration effort. The scale is most often used by people with asthma, or other impaired lung function, which causes the person to become breathless easily. Judge the amount of difficulty you are having with your breathing during exercise according to the following scale:

1. **Mild difficulty:** Noticeable to the exerciser, but not to an observer.

2. **Some difficulty:** Noticeable to an observer.

3. **Moderate difficulty:** Exerciser can still continue.

4. **Severe difficulty:** Exerciser cannot continue.

If you are experiencing severe difficulty, reduce the intensity of the exercise.

that mild shortness of breath is normal when exercising. Be sure to avoid your "trouble zones" by keeping the duration and intensity of your exercise well below those that cause you severe shortness of breath. Monitor your breathing with the Dyspnea Index in this chapter.

Remember that *arm exercises may cause shortness of breath sooner* than leg exercises. Likewise, *cold and dry air can make breathing and exercise more difficult.* This is why swimming can be an especially good activity for chronic lung disease.

If you have severe lung disease. Many people with lung disease believe that it is impossible to exercise, since getting across the room may take a great deal of effort. However, if this sounds like you, exercise is especially important.

Everyone with lung disease who can get out of bed can exercise ten minutes a day. Here is how you do it: Every hour, get up from what you are doing and walk slowly across the room or around your chair for one minute. Doing this ten times a day will add up to ten minutes of exercise. After you have done this for a week or two and are feeling stronger, walk for two minutes every hour. When this feels comfortable (after another week or two), change your pattern to walking three to four minutes at a time every other hour. Again, do this for a week or two, and then try five minutes three or four times a day. Next, try six to eight minutes two or three times a day. Most people with severe lung disease can build up to walking ten to twenty minutes once or twice a day within a few months!

Go slowly. And remember to breathe while exercising.

STROKE   Physical activity, especially physical therapy, is basic in recovery from a person with stroke. Before beginning any conditioning program on your own, check with your doctor to make sure your blood pressure is under control.

If you have weakness or poor balance from your stroke, some activities may cause you to lose your balance, strain, or fall. You may want to use a walker, cane, or "buddy" while you are exercising. You may also wish to sit, or alternate sitting and standing, during your conditioning. If an arm is affected, you may prefer to do leg exercises. If both a leg and an arm are affected, it is probably best to begin with seated exercise. If you already have a prescribed exercise program, talk with your therapist for ideas to combine your therapeutic exercise with a conditioning exercise program.

HYPERTENSION   Before you begin any exercise program, check with your doctor to make sure your blood pressure is under control. This generally means that it is consistently around 160/90 or less. The first blood pressure number (160) is the systolic blood pressure, which normally will go up dur-

Myth: It's dangerous for people with chronic illness to do any exercise.

Fact: Exercise benefits everyone, and it's especially important for people with reduced mobility.

ing vigorous exercise. *If you have hypertension, your systolic blood pressure should never be allowed to go over 200.* The second reading (90) is the diastolic blood pressure, which generally does not increase during exercise.

Avoid exercises that can potentially worsen your hypertension, especially ones that cause you to strain while holding your breath—isometric calisthenics, weight lifting, and rowing, for example—and exercise with arms overhead.

To be safe, you should monitor your own blood pressure at the beginning, middle, and end of your exercise period. You can purchase a blood pressure monitor in most pharmacies, and they are generally easy to use.

If your blood pressure is even higher than 200/110, discontinue your conditioning exercises until you speak with your physician about the need for possible changes in your hypertension treatment plan. For more information, see the chapter Controlling Your Blood Pressure with Exercise.

DIABETES Regular exercise can be a very important part of controlling blood glucose levels and improving health for everyone with diabetes. However, if you are taking medication to control your illness, you should discuss any change in exercise habits with your doctor or nutritionist, since changes in activity levels often require changes in medication and eating schedules.

Mild to moderate aerobic exercise decreases the need for insulin and helps control blood glucose levels by increasing the sensitivity of body cells to insulin and lowering blood glucose levels both during and after exercise. This type of regular exercise also is essential for losing and controlling weight, and for reducing cardiovascular risk factors such as high blood lipid levels and high blood pressure.

The exercise program for diabetics is generally the same as described earlier. The additional considerations of exercise with diabetes are to begin an exercise program only when your diabetes is under good control; keep in touch with your doctor to make changes in medication and diet if needed; and coordinate eating, medication, and exercise to avoid hypoglycemia.

If you have problems with poor circulation, be sure to check your skin regularly and protect yourself from blisters and abrasions. It is especially important to inspect your feet and practice good skin and nail hygiene. Shoe inserts can be made to help protect the soles of the feet.

OSTEOPOROSIS Regular exercise plays an important part in preventing osteoporosis as well as in strengthening bones that already show signs of disease. Weight-bearing aerobic exercise (such as walking and aerobic dance, during which you come down on your feet) and strengthening exercises are the most effective for strengthening bones. Flexibility and back and abdominal strengthening exercises are important for helping maintain good posture. See the aerobics and flexibility chapters, as well as the chapter Keeping Your Back Healthy, for information and exercises.

If you have osteoporosis or think you may be at risk, remember these precautions:

- No heavy lifting.
- Avoid exercises that put you at risk for falls
  (be especially careful on pool decks, icy sidewalks, or waxed floors).

- Never bend over from the waist (such as bending down to touch your toes).

- Don't slouch when doing any exercise—or in every-day life!

- Consider using a cane or walking stick if your balance is poor, when you're in a crowd, or on unfamiliar ground.

RHEUMATOID ARTHRITIS   People with rheumatoid arthritis should pay special attention to flexibility, strengthening, and appropriate use of your joints. Exercises to help maintain joint mobility and attention to good posture will help ease pain and avoid tightness. Be sure to include hand and wrist exercises in your daily program (a good time to do these is during a bath when hands are warm and limber).

Because rheumatoid arthritis sometimes affects the bones in the neck, it is best to avoid extreme neck movements and not to put pressure on the back of the head or neck.

Stiffness in the morning is often a particular problem. Flexibility exercises before getting up or during a hot bath or shower can help. Also, doing gentle flexibility exercises before going to bed in the evening has been shown to reduce morning stiffness.

CLAUDICATION (LEG PAIN)   Exercise for people with claudication in their legs is generally limited only by the leg pain that develops during exercise. Conditioning exercises can help improve endurance and reduce leg pain for most people.

However, if claudication makes it impossible to do any type of leg exercises (thus keeping you from getting the benefit of a conditioning program), bypass surgery on the vessels in the affected leg may be necessary.

To gradually improve endurance and lessen leg pain, perform daily short periods of leg exercise (such as walking or bicycling) just short of the point of leg pain. When discomfort starts, rest or change activities until it subsides. Then repeat the short period of exercise, again to the point of discomfort but not severe pain. Repeat for five to ten minutes at first, and gradually increase it over time to thirty to sixty minutes. Many people find that with this method they can gradually increase the length of time they can walk comfortably.

Remember that arm exercises won't usually cause leg pain, so be sure to include them as an important part of your conditioning program. Also, a method that may help delay calf pain when you walk is to walk more slowly and use more arm swing.

OSTEOARTHRITIS   Since osteoarthritis begins primarily as a problem with joint cartilage, an exercise program should include taking care of cartilage, which needs joint motion and some weight bearing to stay healthy.

Joint cartilage soaks up nutrients and fluid and gets rid of waste products by being squeezed when you move the joint. If the joint is not moved regularly, cartilage deteriorates. If the joint is continually compressed, as the hips and knees are by long periods of standing, the cartilage can't expand and soak up nutrients and fluid.

You should move any joint with osteoarthritis through its full range of motion several time daily. Judge your activity level so pain is not increased.

If hips and knees are involved, limit walking and standing to no more than two to four hours at a time, followed by at least an hour off your feet to give the cartilage time to decompress. Using a cane on the opposite side of a painful hip or knee will reduce joint stress, and often get you over a rough time.

Good posture, strong muscles, and good endurance are important ways to protect cartilage and reduce joint pain.

Good shoes that absorb the stresses of walking are important. Knee-strengthening exercises performed daily can help reduce knee pain and protect the joint.

You're *Never Too Old* to Be Fit

Joyce Adams Hanna, M.A.

The good news is that most things that get worse with aging get better with exercise!

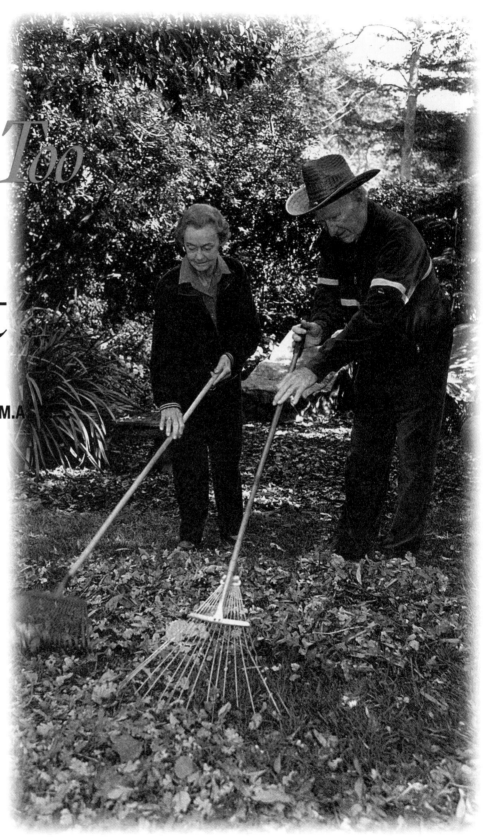

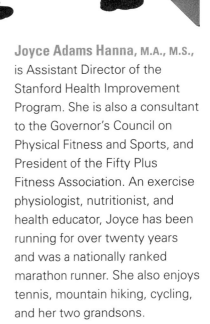

*I*T'S IMPORTANT TO EXERCISE when we're young, but it's imperative to exercise as we get older. Studies increasingly show that as we get older, regular physical activity is a key component to a healthy lifestyle.

Older people who exercise seem to get more enjoyment out of life. They sleep better and wake up with more energy. They maintain their independence longer with a sense of more control over their lives. They are more alert, able to concentrate better, and feel more able to cope with stress. Chronic inactivity is really an abnormal situation to which our human body is not genetically adapted. The National Institute on Aging reports, "If exercise could be packed into a pill, it would be the single most widely prescribed and beneficial medicine in the nation." The good news is that most things that get worse with aging get better with exercise!

Exercise for Good Health

Exercise really can help keep disease from your door. Furthermore, it's never too late to begin reducing your risk. More and more studies indicate that physical activity can help reduce our risk for colon cancer, breast cancer, and prostate cancer. The American Heart Association has recently identified lack of physical activity as one of the four major risk factors for heart disease (along with high cholesterol, high blood pressure, and smoking). We know now that physical activity has a unique influence, independent of other risk factors, on reducing risk for disease and prolonging life.

Studies show that physical activity helps reduce our risk for osteoporosis, a disease that affects one out of four post-

Joyce Adams Hanna, M.A., M.S., is Assistant Director of the Stanford Health Improvement Program. She is also a consultant to the Governor's Council on Physical Fitness and Sports, and President of the Fifty Plus Fitness Association. An exercise physiologist, nutritionist, and health educator, Joyce has been running for over twenty years and was a nationally ranked marathon runner. She also enjoys tennis, mountain hiking, cycling, and her two grandsons.

menopausal women. When we do weight-bearing activities, such as walking, we apply stress to the bone, which helps maintain and build bone density. New studies are showing that resistance or strength training can increase bone density—at any age—as well as increase muscle strength and balance. This increase in strength and balance is important because it decreases our liklihood for falling, which is the greatest risk for fractures in older people.

Our bodies are much more pliable than we previously suspected. No matter what our age, our arteries, muscles, and bones have a tremendous ability to adapt and become healthier with a more active lifestyle.

Studies on exercise and aging increasingly show the life-extending power of regular exercise. More important, perhaps, is that quality of life is also enhanced. Recent data from a long-term study indicate that even modest amounts of exercise can substantially reduce our likelihood of dying from heart disease, cancer, and other causes. (See the box "A Long and Healthy Life: The Harvard Alumni Study" in this chapter.)

Here's the most striking—and encouraging—finding: The biggest health gains come from people just moving out of the most sedentary category into the moderate exercise category. For example, going from being sedentary to walking briskly for half an hour on most days can drop your risk for disease dramatically over a period of time. This means that important health benefits are within almost everybody's reach.

Another long-term study showed that middle-aged and elderly men (between forty-five and eight-four years old) who took up moderately vigorous activities like brisk walking or swimming have a 23 to 29 percent lower overall death rate

How Much Exercise Is Enough?

There is no particular magic to the figure of 2,000 kcal. Any activity (even one that burns as little as 500 kcal a week) is better than none, and the benefits will increase steadily up to a level of about 3,500 kcal a week, and possibly much further. Even if you spent the rest of the day in bed, you would burn 2,000 kcal through any of the following activities, in any combination that you wanted:

- 57 minutes a day of light sports play
- 35 minutes a day of moderate sports play
- 28 minutes a day of vigorous sports play
- 2¾ miles of walking a day
- Climbing up and down 800 steps a day (about 40 stories of a modern office building)

Even if you already maintain a high level of exercise by climbing stairs or walking, there is certainly no reason to exclude sports. In general, our study and others have found that the more activity you can include in your life, the better.

than nonexercisers, and up to a 14 percent reduction in the risk of coronary artery disease. One of the most exciting results of this study was that even men who waited until they were over sixty-five to begin moderate exercise gained in life expectancy. The apparent life extension may not be long for an elderly person, maybe a year or two, but the other benefits of improved quality of life and freedom from disease are major gains. One of the positive associations we can make with exercise and longevity is focusing not on postponing death but on maintaining health and vitality for the longest period of our lives.

Functional Health: Living Well

An active lifestyle, particularly one that includes some weight-bearing activities, protects us against limitations in our functional health status. *Functional health* is our ability to perform the usual activities of daily life—bathing, dressing, preparing

A Long and Healthy Life: The Harvard Alumni Study

Ralph S. Paffenbarger, Jr., M.D., DR. P.H.

Exercise not only enhances quality of life, it actually prolongs life. To understand how and why, we'll look at the results of a study involving nearly 17,000 male Harvard alumni over three decades.

Our observations began in the early 1960s. At the core of this survey were questions designed to measure the men's current levels of physical activity. They were asked to report how far they walked in an average day, how many flights of stairs they climbed, and what type and amount of sports play they regularly engaged in, including gardening and work around the house or garage.

On the basis of their reports, we then computed the total amount of energy that each man expended each week in terms of the number of kilocalories (kcal) used up at the following rate:

- stair-climbing: 40 kcal per 100 steps, up and down
- walking: 100 kcal per mile (twelve blocks)
- light sports: 5 kcal per minute
- moderate sports: 8 kcal per minute
- heavy sports: 10 kcal per minute

We also inquired about their state of health, including questions on smoking and drinking patterns, family health history, and specific chronic diseases, such as hypertension (high blood pressure). We also checked their student health and athletic records to find out their state of health as freshmen and whether or not they had participated in varsity or intramural sports during their four years in college.

Some 20,000 alumni furnished us with the information we had requested. Excluding about 3,000 (who had evidence of coronary heart disease at the beginning of the study), we have been following their progress ever since.

EXERCISE HELPS CUT OTHER RISKS

What did we find? The short answer is that regular exercise did indeed reduce the risk of premature death considerably. Those who expended 2,000 kcal or more a week in exercise had a rate of premature death from all causes that was 28 percent less than that of their sedentary counterparts in a sixteen-year follow-up period. *This translates into one to two years or more of extra life.*

Heart disease. The reduction in heart disease accounts for most of the difference in premature death between the active men and the sedentary men. This was apparent in all groups of exercisers, including those whose risk was elevated by other risk factors such as smoking, high blood pressure, and a family history of short survival.

Cigarette smoking. For example, we found that cigarette smoking increased the risk of coronary heart disease considerably. If none of the alumni had smoked cigarettes, the death rate from heart disease would have been 25 percent lower in these sixteen years.

When you add exercise to the equation, the risk was reduced significantly. A moderate smoker (up to a pack a day) who expended 2,000 kcal a week in exercise would still have more risk of heart disease than a nonsmoker;

but his risk would be about half that of a moderate smoker who had little or no exercise.

High blood pressure. We made a similar observation for hypertension. While high blood pressure in general increased risk by 118 percent, much of this extra risk could be offset by exercise. Hypertensives who expended more than 2,000 kcal a week in exercise had less than half the death rate from cardiovascular disease of their sedentary contemporaries.

Family history of heart disease. Parental history of heart disease provides an even more striking example. A sedentary man with cardiovascular disease on both sides of his family doubles his own risk of coronary heart disease. But an active man with the same family history who expended at least 2,000 kcal a week would essentially *neutralize* his genetic risk. Indeed, his risk would be lower than that of a sedentary man with no heart disease in his family.

ACTIVE PEOPLE ARE HEALTHIER

As you weigh the benefits of exercise, you may be pondering two questions: Are people healthy because they exercise, or do they exercise because they are healthy? Generally speaking, people do not exercise because they are healthy; they are healthy because they exercise. A number of facts support this contention:

1. The association between exercise and reduced risk of coronary heart disease is strong and consistent—regardless of age, race, or sex.

2. Exercise makes an independent contribution to the delay of coronary heart disease and to the prolongation of life, whether or not a person smokes, has high blood pressure, is obese, or has weight that goes up and down. The benefit of exercise is independent from adverse family history, from high or low cholesterol, and from abnormal glucose metabolism.

3. The relation between exercise and risk of coronary heart disease is persistent in successive increments of time—that is, what is true for, say, three years will remain true for the next three years, and the next.

With all this, it makes common sense to believe that exercise can increase life expectancy and delay disease. And you don't have to spend those extra years doing nothing but jogging. Our calculations show that a forty-year-old man who exercises for three hours a week, with a total expenditure of 2,000 kcal each week, will earn more extra life than the time he spends exercising: For each hour of exercise, he can expect 1.95 hours more life than his sedentary counterpart.

Ralph S. Paffenbarger, Jr., M.D., DR. P.H., is Professor of Epidemiology, Stanford University School of Medicine, and Adjunct Professor of Epidemiology of the Harvard University School of Public Health. He has completed eighteen Boston marathons and five Western States 100-mile runs, and currently enjoys brisk walking.

> "It's never too late to be fit. If ninety-year-olds who never exercised can start a weight-lifting program and become more fit—and they can—you can too."
>
> —Terrie Rizzo

meals, shopping, and all the rest. This becomes more and more important to our self-esteem and self-efficacy—our sense of self-mastery—as we move into our later years.

People who are more active are less likely to decline functionally as they get older. Data show that a sixty-five-year-old man who is physically active has the functional capacity of a forty-year-old man who is sedentary. That means that active people are physiologically about twenty years younger than their sedentary friends. This is an outstanding advantage. It means many more disability-free days to meet and enjoy responsibilities and activities, thus giving an active older person a higher quality of life.

Exercise Helps Control Weight

As we grow older, many of us complain that we are gaining weight while eating the same amounts, or even eating less. Part of the reason for this frustrating dilemma is that most people become less physically active as they get older and simply burn fewer calories over a twenty-four-hour period. The cumulative effect of even a small change in physical activity plays an important role in weight control over a period of time.

A larger part of the weight problem as we get older, however, is due to changes in body composition. The average American loses approximately 6.6 pounds of muscle mass from young adulthood into middle age. Then, at around age forty-five, the rate of loss speeds up. Since muscle is active tissue, it requires more calories to sustain itself than fat tissue. The more muscle our body has, the faster our metabolism will be—the calories needed by the body just to sustain itself. Therefore the more muscle we have, the more calories we will burn on a daily basis, and the more successful we will be at controlling our weight at a healthy level.

Most of this decline in muscle mass and metabolism is *not* inevitable as we get older. We can counteract this tendency with an active lifestyle, regular exercise, and some strength training (for details, see the chapter Using Your Muscles for Life).

Use It or Lose It

We know now that many of the changes that we have previously ascribed to the normal aging process are, in fact, caused by lack of activity or disuse. Physical activity has *something* in it for everybody, and it has almost *everything* in it for the older person.

Older adults can receive tremendous benefits from physical activity. Regular exercise helps decrease:

- body fat percentage
- bone loss
- resting heart rate
- falls and fractures
- blood pressure
- anxiety and depression
- risk of heart attack (both initial and subsequent)
- stress
- frailty and disability in older years
- triglycerides
- blood glucose

Regular exercise helps increase:

Myth: The older you are, the less exercise you need.

Fact: Exercise is important when you're young, and it's imperative when you get older. After forty, we're too old not to exercise!

Myth: It's not important to do weight (strength) training when you get older.

Fact: Actually, strength training is one of the most important steps in slowing down the aging process. It has a positive influence on bone density, metabolism, body fat percentage, and balance —all elements of a healthy, active life.

- lean muscle mass

- strength

- metabolic rate

- aerobic capacity

- bone density

- flexibility

- self-esteem

- self-efficacy (a sense of self-mastery)

- quality of sleep

- HDL (good cholesterol)

- balance

- functional health status

- blood-sugar tolerance

- quality of life

- reaction time

- ability to regulate internal body temperature

- high-quality longevity

With every good reason to begin exercising, why not get started today? When you're planning your activity program, remember to balance it by including exercises in the following four areas: (1) lifestyle activity, (2) cardiovascular endurance, (3) muscle strength, and (4) flexibility. The rest of this chapter gives you some good ideas that you can implement to begin exercising—right now!

Part 1: Lifestyle Activity

Remember that doing something is better than doing nothing! People who do a little bit of exercise are better off than people who do none. Think of it this way: Sitting is better than lying down, standing is better than sitting, moving around is better than standing, and brisk walking is better than just moving around.

If you are presently sedentary, aim for being a little less sedentary each day—five minutes here and ten minutes there add up to quite a bit of activity over the course of a day. Your possibilities are unlimited: Get up and move around during TV commercials, rake leaves in your yard, use the stairs instead of the elevator, wash your car, take up an active hobby like square dancing, walk part of the way to and from work, or walk to do short errands. Look for opportunities to expend more energy that fits into your particular lifestyle. These short lifestyle activities can have an important cumulative effect in your overall level of activity and health.

GETTING STARTED The following guidelines will help you as you begin to become more active:

1. If you are not doing any physical activity right now, begin by adding a few minutes of increased activity into your day.

2. Build up gradually to thirty minutes of accumulated physical activity on most days.

3. If all your activities are at a fairly low level, aim for accumulating more than thirty minutes a day.

It's a good idea to have more than one aerobic activity. If you're ready to add more exercise to your program, here are some other ideas:

- low-impact aerobic dance
- treadmill walking
- hiking
- race walking or power walking
- backpacking
- tennis
- rowing
- cycling (stationary and road)
- kayaking and canoeing
- stair stepping
- square and ballroom dancing
- water aerobics
- swimming
- cross-country skiing

Part 2: Cardiovascular Endurance

It's also beneficial to include some specific cardiovascular exercise sessions in your week. Your program should include a planned thirty- to forty-five-minute brisk exercise or recreation session three or four times a week. There are many activities that build your cardiovascular endurance.

Walking is one of the easiest activities because you can do it almost everywhere, and the only equipment you need is a good pair of walking shoes. It's also one of the best: Walking involves several major muscle groups and puts very little strain on the joints. Many people find that walking two miles briskly on most days of the week is an enjoyable way to get their exercise.

The American College of Sports Medicine and American Heart Association guidelines indicate that the great majority of apparently healthy adults can start an exercise program with minimal medical screening. Almost everybody can walk for health and fitness!

GETTING STARTED   The following guidelines will help you enjoy your walking and reduce your risk of injury:

1. Set aside a specific time of day to walk. Choose a time when you are usually not tired. Walking with music or a friend or a group can add interest and variety to your program.

2. Walk only if you are feeling well. Don't try to exercise through a cold, flu, or other illness. When you are feeling better, return to your program.

3. Wear loose comfortable clothing and supportive shoes that fit well.

4. Before starting your walk, warm up the muscles you will be using by doing a few gentle calisthenics.

5. Gently stretch your muscles (no bouncing) after warming up.

6. Walk within your comfort range. Walking should not cause pain or stiffness, nor should it make you feel breathless or off balance.

7. If you are feeling tired two hours after you are finished walking, slow down in your next workout. Walking should leave you feeling invigorated, not exhausted.

8. If you've been sedentary, start with five- to ten-minute walks every other day. Increase your exercise time by five to ten minutes each week.

9. Try to work up to a thirty-minute walk on most days. If you can't manage a thirty-minute session, try three ten-minute walks a day.

10. Your long-term goal could be to walk one to three miles in thirty to forty-five minutes.

11. After walking, stretch your muscles again for five to ten minutes.

12. Remember to drink plenty of water before, during, and after exercise.

13. If you have problems such as dizziness, chest discomfort, shortness of breath, or leg pain, consult your physician.

Part 3. Muscle Strength

Studies show that one of the most critical steps in slowing down the aging process is strength training, also called resistance or weight training. As we get older, the average person—who is not exercising—starts losing muscle mass, and the rate of this loss can increase after age forty-five. The exciting news is that people at any age, even the frail elderly, can increase their muscle mass and their strength.

Maintenance of muscle mass and strength can have important positive influences on our bone density, balance, resting metabolism, and body fat percentage, plus a host of other benefits that increase quality of life. We know enough now to state that there is no reason for strength to belong just to the young. The benefits of strength training are available to all of us at any time of our life.

Strength training can consist of any exercise that builds strength by working your muscles against resistance. This can be done by using hand and leg weights or special kinds of rubber bands that you can buy at a sporting goods store. You don't need to buy weights, however, to do resistance training at home. You can make excellent weights out of plastic water, milk, or detergent jugs with handles. Partially fill the jugs with sand or water to a point where you can lift them fairly easily. Weigh your homemade weights on your bathroom scale. As you get stronger, you can add more water or sand to increase the weight.

You also can do your strength training in a weight room with a variety of weight training equipment. It's important to have a qualified person show you how to use the equipment safely and effectively. For many people, strength training can begin with pushing against the weight of their own bodies without any equipment. Sit-ups and push-ups are examples of using your own weight as resistance. Before starting a resistance program, older people should check with their physician to find out whether any special cautions apply to their situation.

GETTING STARTED   The following guidelines will help you get stronger, make the exercises more enjoyable, and reduce your risk of injury.

1.   Try to do some strength training two to three nonconsecutive days a week. Plan your routine to avoid exercising the same muscle two times in a row. For example, you might want to work your legs on Tuesday and your upper body on Thursday.

2.   Before starting your resistance exercises, warm up the muscles you will be using by doing some gentle calisthenics or brisk walking for five to ten minutes.

3.   Gently stretch your muscles (no bouncing) after your warm-up.

4.   Start your strength training in your comfort range. Begin with low weights—somewhere between one to five pounds. Begin with a weight that you can lift ten times. If you can do more than twenty lifts, the weight is too light.

5.   Lift the weight in a slow, controlled fashion, taking six to nine seconds to lift it through the entire range of motion. Don't swing a weight rapidly or bounce at the end of the movement. Concentrate on each muscle group as you work on it.

6.   It's important to breathe correctly when lifting weights: Inhale before lifting, then exhale while lifting, and inhale

Myth: Exercise puts stress on my bones.

Fact: Exercise is *good* for your bones! Weight-bearing activities—walking, climbing stairs, dancing, and strength training—all build and maintain bone density.

again as you slowly return to the starting position. Never hold your breath while lifting.

7. Train only in the range of motion where you have no pain. If it hurts, don't do it!

8. Rest a few seconds between each lift.

9. The appropriate amount of weight for you to do your strength training is the amount you can lift between eight and twelve times, after which your muscles should be too tired to continue. As you get stronger, you may be able to do two or three sets for each exercise.

10. Increase the resistance gradually, trying to lift a little more weight a few more times each week, but do not increase the weight or number of lifts more than once a week. If you have to hold your breath to lift, you are probably using too much weight.

11. Listen to your body. Some days you will feel stronger than others. Adjust your work with your weights accordingly.

12. Following your workout, slowly stretch each muscle group for five to ten minutes.

Part 4: Flexibility

Flexibility refers to the ability of the joints to move freely and without pain or stiffness through a wide range of motion. This ability means that the muscles around the joints be stretched regularly. Flexibility varies from person to person and from joint to joint. Good flexibility is thought to protect the muscles against injury, since flexible muscles are actually longer and less likely to "tear" and "pull" than inflexible ones.

Myth: I have to do activities like jog or take an aerobics class to get any benefit from exercise.

Fact: You can also achieve benefits to your overall health by accumulating thirty minutes or more of moderate intensity physical activity over the course of the day. Walking your dog, ballroom dancing, gardening for eight to ten minutes or longer can all contribute to the thirty-minute total.

Flexibility is also important in helping us perform daily tasks that involve moving objects, reaching, and twisting and turning our body. As we get older, the tissues around our joints tend to thicken and become less pliable. Muscles may grow shorter and range of motion decreases. Gentle stretching exercises are the best way to combat these tendencies. There is plenty of evidence that flexibility can be improved at any age.

Swimming, water activities, gentle ballet, and yoga programs specifically designed for older adults are all excellent activities for increasing flexibility. A gentle, overall stretching program is an important part of managing arthritis and osteoporosis. A stretching program can also help keep your hamstrings (the back of the thigh) and hips flexible—key elements in decreasing risk of low back pain.

GETTING STARTED The following guidelines will help you increase your flexibility and reduce your risk of injury:

1. Try to do some gentle stretching every day. Stretch your muscles before and after your strength workout. Include some stretching as part of your cardiovascular workout.

2. Warm up before stretching with about five minutes of walking or gentle calisthenics. Your tissues will lengthen more easily when they are warm.

3. Gently and slowly ease into each stretch in a controlled manner (no bouncing), until you can just feel the muscle stretch. Do not force the stretch. Hold the position in a relaxed manner ten to twenty seconds, relax, and repeat.

4. It's important to breathe naturally and regularly dur-

If You Have Concerns About Your Health

If you have symptoms that need to be checked out, or if you have a chronic disease, see your doctor and have a thorough medical evaluation before you begin an exercise program. You might need more specific exercise recommendations than we can provide here. If you answer yes to any of the items on the Physical Activity Readiness Questionnaire (in the chapter Don't Hurt Yourself!), we recommend that you consult with your personal physician before increasing your physical activity.

ing your stretch workout. "Breathe into" each muscle group as you stretch it. Never hold your breath while stretching.

5. If a stretch hurts, stop doing it. Make stretching a relaxing, pleasurable part of you program. Listen to your body and avoid doing anything that causes pain.

It's Never Too Late to Start!

Getting older means something very different today than even a few decades ago. Americans are rethinking their old preconceptions about aging, and creating a new image—one that's full of vitality, strength, and active living. It's clear that an active lifestyle with a physical activity program can have a dynamic impact on our health and well-being. Physical activity can be a potent catalyst in helping us reach the ideal: A health span that keeps up with our life span. No matter what your age, it's never too late to start exercising!

Notes

CHAPTER 5. *Mind + Body: The No-Stress Equation*

1. The seated exercises in this chapter are taken from the registered, copyrighted program Sittercise™. A brochure of the complete series of thirty-six seated exercises is available from the Stanford Health Promotion Resource Center, 1000 Welch Road, Palo Alto, CA 94304. For pricing and ordering information, call (415) 723-7049.

2. If you would like to learn more about the complex underlying science and neurophysiology of the mind-body approach to relaxation, see Ken Pelletier, *Mind as Healer, Mind as Slayer* (1992); and Ken Pelletier, *Sound Mind, Sound Body* (New York: Simon & Schuster, 1995).

CHAPTER 15. *Customizing Exercise for Special Needs*

1. For more information on this subject, see Kate Lorig, M.D., *et al., Living a Healthy Life with Chronic Conditions* (Palo Alto, CA: Bull Publishing Company, 1994); and Kate Lorig and Jonathan Fries, *The Arthritis Helpbook* (Reading, MA: Addison-Wesley Publishing Company, 1995).

Many thanks for the donation of time on the part of the following people who were photographed for the part, and chapter opening pages: p. i: Terrie Heinrich Rizzo, Manager of Health and Fitness Education Programs, Stanford Health Improvement Program. **p. ii:** Jeff Petry, Computer Systems Manager, SCRDP. **p. iii:** Jerrie Moo-Thurman, Fitness Coordinator, Stanford Health Improvement Program. **p. vii:** Dave Ahn, Senior Applications Software Developer, Research/Instructional Applications, SCRDP. **p. viii:** Joyce Adams Hanna, Assistant Director, Stanford Health Improvement Program. **p. ix:** Tony Thurman, affiliated with the Stanford Health Improvement Program. **p. x:** Elizabeth Wright, Exercise Physiologist, Stanford Health Improvement Program. **pp xvi-1:** Terrie Heinrich Rizzo. **p. 2:** John Castillo (left) and Chip Cullison (right), both affiliated with the Health Improvement Program. **p. 13:** Catherine O'Brien, Director of the Stanford Video Media Group, and Sugar. **p. 30:** Yosuke Chikamoto, Manager of Research and Development, Stanford Health Improvement Program. **p. 43:** Kim Bluitt, Stanford Class of '92, Program Director, Alumni Relations, Stanford Alumni Association. **pp. 58-59:** Stanford employees from a variety of departments participating in the Health Improvement Program's Healthy Back/Strong Abs class. **p. 60:** Karl Garcia, Stanford Class of '85. **p. 72:** Stanford employees from the Operations and Maintainence Department participating in the regular noon basketball game. **p. 88:** Regina Rebosura, Distribution Center Assistant, Stanford Health Promotion Resouce Center. **p. 112:** Terrie Rizzo assisting Pamela Perkins (on mat), Director of Development for Stanford Health Services. **pp. 125, 139, 158:** Terrie Heinrich Rizzo. **pp. 182–183:** Stanford employees from a variety of departments participating in the Health Improvement Program's Water Aerobics class. **p. 184:** Margaret Vorse Thompson (left), Stanford Class of '51. Nancy Thompson Nichols (right), Director of Professional Education, Stanford Alumni Association. **p. 189:** Elaine Tencati, Research Assistant/Technical Assistance Coordinator, SCRDP. **p. 200:** Ann Hamon (left), Administrative Associate, SCRDP. Barbara Jackson (right), Group Leader, Stanford Chronic Disease Self-Management Course. **p. 218:** Edna and William "Dutch" Fehring, retired Head Coach of the Stanford Baseball Team.

*I*ndex

Support your local public broadcasting station!

Every community across America is reached by one of the 346 member stations of the Public Broadcasting Service. These stations bring information, entertainment, and insight for the whole family.

Think about the programs you enjoy and remember most:

Masterpiece Theatre. . . Mystery!. . . Nova. . . Nature. . . Sesame Street. . . Ghostwriter. . . Reading Rainbow. . . Baseball. . . The Civil War. . . The American Experience. . . The News Hour with Jim Lehrer. . . Great Performances. . . Washington Week in Review. . . and so many more.

On your local PBS station, you'll also find fascinating adult education courses, provocative documentaries, great cooking and do-it-yourself programs, and thoughtful local analysis.

Despite the generous underwriting contributions of foundations and corporations, more than half of all public television budgets come from individual member support.

For less than the cost of a night at the movies, less than a couple of months of a daily paper, less than a month of your cable TV bill, you can help make possible all the quality programming you enjoy.

Become a member of your public broadcasting station and do your part.

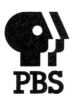 **Public Television. You make it happen!**